THE HUMAN
MACHINE

A TROUBLE-SHOOTER'S MANUAL
VOLUME III

Hiatal Hernia Syndrome Epidemic

FROM INDIGESTION TO ACHES AND PAINS TO
DEGENERATIVE CONDITIONS TO CANCER

PHIL SELINSKY, N.D.

Box 191
Santa Barbara, California 93102
(805) 963-5005
(626) 963-5023
909-741-7582 FAX
e-mail <ihss@earthlink.net>
Web site <thehumanmachine.com>
Second printing 2018

ISBN Softcover   978-1-950580-74-3

This text was authored to assist students and clients to understand how and why dis-ease occurs and what remedies are available. This information is offered for educational purposes.

No "medical advice" is either expressed or implied...

I TEACH HEALTH,
I DO NOT TREAT DISEASE!

Printed in the United States of America.

To order additional copies of this book, contact:
Bookwhip
1-855-339-3589
https://www.bookwhip.com

Table of Contents

Forward

Phil Selinsky, a doctor of naturopathic medicine makes his medical skills available to the residents of the great state of California and beyond.

His current publication, "The Human Machine … A Trouble Shooter's Manual" brings attention to alternative methods and solutions for many different disease conditions. His approach, whereas novel, is superior in many respects to current, conventional methods of treating medical problems.

In a world where over-medication is so highly prevalent, often to the detriment of the patient's health status, alternative approaches to healthcare must be explored and instituted, particularly when proven, measurable benefits result. Unfortunately, we live in a climate where healthcare is largely controlled by insurance companies, governments, pharmaceutical manufacturers, etc.

Dr. Selinsky's methods are dedicated to the patient's welfare, a move in the right direction. In view of this, his approaches should be more widely implemented and he should receive appropriate recognition and support for his work.

- Fred Kahn, MD, FRCS(C) -

Acknowledgements

First, I would like to acknowledge and express my appreciation for the gene patterns that I inherited from my parents, Oliver and Ann (Gailiusis) Selinsky, that have enabled me to gather the knowledge and expertise to write this book series. Without their collective and combined gene traits and up-bringing environment, with all the pertinent challenges that they provided, I would not have been able to present the perspective on life that I have acquired. I feel very fortunate and grateful for the opportunity to have gone through my "conditioning years" with my parents. Yes we experienced a few challenging and stressful years, but I made it through and I'd like to share a few of my insights with anyone who will listen.

Next I would like to express my gratitude to all of my immediate family and friends and clients who have supported and encouraged my efforts to get this information out of my head and into a format that can be passed to others. Your guidance and personal information helped to write this book series. You have been my very own personal "lab rats and gurus" who, over the years, have taught me how to "listen" and apply the universal principles of physics to all aspects of life.

And of course none of this book series would ever have been completed without the genius and graphic expertise of Edward Layola. I had been looking for years for someone who could look into my brain and "copy and paste" it onto paper. I would tell him what I want to see and he would pull it out of his computer just like I saw in my brain. He is truly an artist with the computer. Also I owe gratitude to Eva Silberman who added her artistic talents to the "body" drawings in this book.

I would also like to acknowledge all the tech support and marketing information given by numerous individuals over the years.

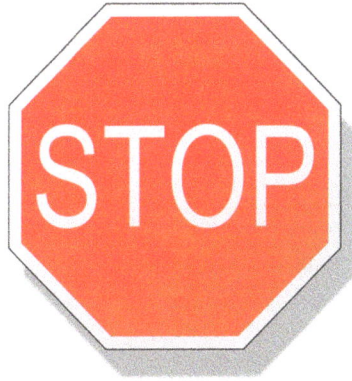

If you are not ready and willing to take the
responsibility for your own health, then

Put This Book Down!

This is <u>not</u> another "take this for that" book.

This is an Owner's Manual.

In this book series you will learn how and why
your vehicle (your body) works.

You will learn how to read the "dash board gages"
on your vehicle (sore spots).

You will learn that pain means that something
is out of balance.

In this Third Volume of the series, you will see
how a genetic defect in your "parts"
can result in a multitude of dis – ease symptoms.

PART I

INTRODUCTION AND PURPOSE

This is an opportunity for Sheople

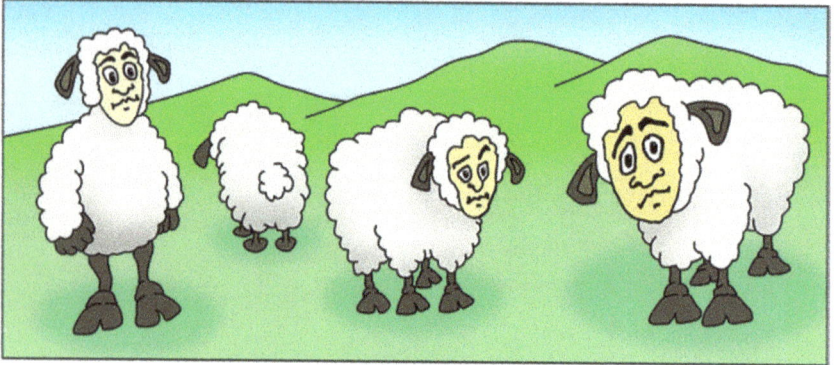

to become People.

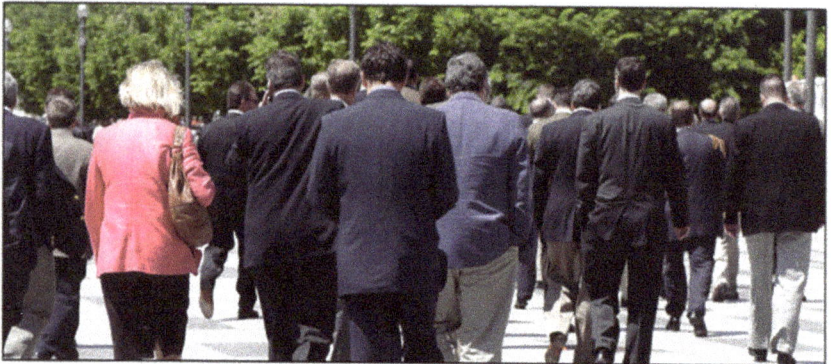

It only takes a few barking dogs to control the herd.

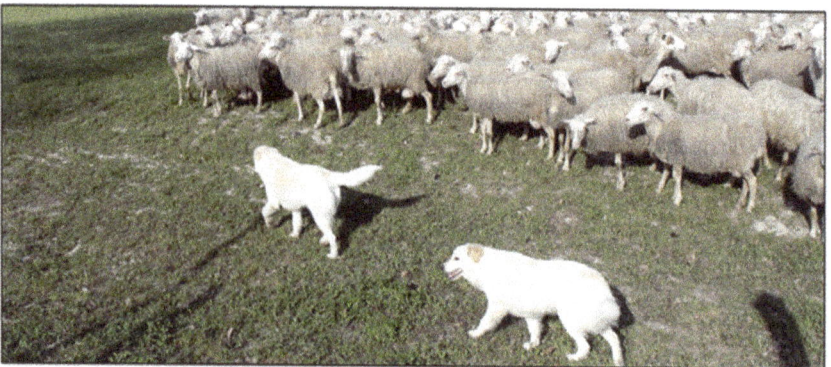

Sheople

The word "**sheople**" or "sheeple" has been used recently to describe humans who are blindly and emotionally herded into or from a belief or practice or custom by a few loud and persistent voices. In Volume II of this series, I discuss the difference between freedom (leading to responsibility) and security (leading to total dependence). I make the statement that:

> "**With total Security you have no Freedom. Conversely, with total Freedom, you have no Security.**" **And along with total Freedom comes total responsibility.**

The vast majority of "**sheople**" feel secure in the herd. And the herd is easily frightened and controlled by a few barking dogs … a few loud and persistent voices who have an agenda that is most times beneficial to the owners of the barking dogs and to the ultimate detriment of the masses (the herd).

The sheep are controlled and herded into pens by the dogs so that the owners can harvest the wool from the sheep. The sheep have no clue that they are being cared for and controlled so that they can be sheared on a regular basis.

Sheople, in general, have no clue that they are being "cared for" and controlled by "owners" so that they can be regularly "sheared". Big corporations take more and more profits and governments take more and more taxes from the **sheople** regularly by convincing the **sheople** that everything is done for the "good" and security of all. The greatest danger to the health of the **sheople** is the corporate agri-business and pharmaceutical industry. Please do a Google search on Edward L. Bernays … the father of spin and crowd control.

A few **sheople** are waking up and becoming **people** who are willing to take responsibility for their ultimate health and wellbeing. They are realizing that pain and discomfort can be avoided by breaking away from the herd mentality. This concept applies to the "alternative" as well as the conventional (allopathic) approach to pain and misery.

Preface

In my Naturopathic practice over the years I have found myself repeating the same stories and lessons that I have learned over and over again until I could tell them in my sleep. So in the interest of preserving my vocal chords and taking advantage of the opportunity to reach many more people with the same or similar problems, I have written a book.

As a matter of fact, I have written a three-book series explaining some of my discoveries over the years that shed some light on the reasons that this Human Machine behaves the way it does. (See "WHAT I'VE LEARNED on page 19.

This book series goes past the typical attempt to suggest remedies for a plethora of symptoms and conditions that plague the human race with pain and discomforts of all sorts.

In this book series, I will try to show that attempting to micromanage this machine with drugs and supplements is typically a total waste of time and resources ... *and it's a dangerous practice.*

If we just learn to understand what the body is trying to accomplish or attempting to balance when it appears to malfunction, and if we can read and understand the "dashboard gages", bells, and whistles (aches and pains), we should on average have a fairly pleasant experience here in our bodies.

This book series is an engineer's perspective on how machines are designed and built to function and to serve humans.

THIS "HUMAN MACHINE" IS NO EXCEPTION

Volume I of **THE HUMAN MACHINE ... A TROUBLE SHOOTER'S MANUAL** explains some of the structural and conditioning influences that shape our view of life and consequently our behavior in society, which usually creates conflicts, which creates stress, which results in **dis – ease** of some sort.

Volume II describes how blood chemistry drives our behavior, within our structural capacity, of course. It also shows how and why we develop conditions of **dis – ease** that are due to *distortions of our **blood chemistry***. We can then easily see how balancing blood chemistry through "proper" nutrition takes the pain away.

This **Volume III** focuses on the physical *distortions (both genetic and traumatic), of the organs of the digestive system* starting with the **Hiatal Hernia Syndrome** involving the stomach. This stomach trauma results in small and large intestine malfunction, which affects nutrient <u>absorption</u>, and creates toxic overload, which leads to **dis – ease** profiles that cause most of all the common aches and pains in our lives.

Theodore Baroody, N.D., D.C., PhD., wrote an excellent book on what he calls "A Guide to Self-Healing of **Hiatal Hernia**". He also wrote books on nutrition especially on the subject of acid/alkaline balance in the blood.

George Goodheart, D.C. is considered the "father" of what is termed "Applied Kinesiology". He developed the practice of testing the relative strength of muscles in the body to determine the correlation between neurological assessment of spinal stresses and acupuncture meridian imbalances.

Fred Stoner, D.C. wrote "The Eclectic Approach to Chiropractic", expanding on Goodheart's discoveries. He was a driving force behind the ICAK (International College of Applied Kinesiology), an organization of medical professionals.

John Thie, D.C. established his claim to fame with his internationally acclaimed book, "Touch for Health", also based on the discoveries of Goodheart and geared more toward the layman.

Each of these brilliant individuals, along with a multitude of researchers and scientists has alluded to the fact that "energy" drives this body. They've had the keys in their hands all along, but have not yet turned the key in the lock. Each one has described how to alleviate pain using acupuncture/acupressure points and adding certain dietary supplements. But no one yet has spelled out the mechanical connections between the "energy" and the structure/function of the body and WHY pain develops when "energy" is distorted.

This book series will explain in simple terms what the connection of all the parts is supposed to accomplish. This HUMAN MACHINE (our physical body) has a specific design purpose and follows all the laws of physics as it attempts to carry you (Consciousness) from the beginning of your experience here on planet Earth to the last moment of your sojourn, no matter how long or short that period of time may be.

Western Allopathic Medicine and Traditional Chinese Medicine appear to approach dis – ease (disease) from a slightly different perspective. In this book series, I will attempt to translate between Eastern and Western concepts and philosophies. I will show that both approaches attempt to say the same things in different languages.

Just sit back, relax, and picture yourself literally driving and steering this Human Machine (body) through the highway of life … always with one eye on the "dashboard gages", watching and listening for strange sensations and noises that might alert you to a possible present or future problem.

It's not that difficult. *To experience a "smooth ride", you have to know the design limitations and the proper fuel for your own model vehicle and you must also undergo regular maintenance procedures and inspections.*

And always remember …

PAIN RESULTS FROM THE VIOLATION OF THE LAWS OF PHYSICS

You Don't "Mess" With Mother Nature Without Paying a Price.

Introduction

There are two issues that I should address before I present the information in this book.

Issue #1: People over the years have asked me about the motivating force that changed my focus from mechanical engineering to human health concerns. "What's the connection between steel and plastic machine design engineering and flesh and blood machine design engineering?"

Issue #2: My mother died on November 15, 2010. She made it to just a few weeks shy of 99.

Why is this information important to discuss?

What is the connection between these two issues?

Answer to #1: Physics ... the laws of physics apply equally to steel and plastic machines as well as flesh and blood machines including all forms of life here on this planet. Relating the laws of physics (from my engineering background) to the physical challenges that I experienced in my early years, I now understand that almost all of my physical problems could have been avoided if my parents knew then what I know now.

Answer to #2: While she was alive my mother was very alert and aware of current affairs and current political chicanery. She stayed up to date on life around her. She would have read my material for sure.

CONNECTING ISSUE #1 WITH ISSUE #2

Now that my mother is gone, I can freely analyze and back- engineer and disclose in print what happened to my body in my younger years now without fear of her feeling guilty because of her ignorance at the time. If she read this material, I know she would anguish over feeling responsible for the things that happened to my body. So now I can tell …

My Story

I'm the eldest of 7 children. We grew up at the end of a dirt road on the outskirts of northwest Detroit that at that time was called Southfield Township. Zip codes were not invented yet. Our mailing address was Detroit 19, Michigan. Our "party-line" phone number was "Southfield 3244".

I mention these details just to give a little flavor to the fact that we lived meagerly without a lot of frills. My parents did all that they knew how to do at the time to see that all of us kids had what we needed to make it to adulthood without too many dents and dings.

In my case I had a few out-of-the-ordinary challenges along the way. I doubt that what I had experienced was all that different from most other kids, but looking back now, I can see WHY things happened the way they did.

I have "back-engineered" my past experiences and can now easily explain the mechanics and the physics behind all the health difficulties that took place.

My hope is that my sharing this information on my shortcomings might help others to make their lives and that of their family more comfortable and pain free.

In addition to going through all the usual childhood diseases, I had a couple of "extras" that I would like to share with you here that might help you to think about your own life and health issues and that of your children.

As I mentioned, with 7 hungry growing kids to feed there weren't too many available choices for good wholesome food. We ate a lot of filler type foods like macaroni and white bread and spaghetti and hamburger and kool-aid ... with lots of sugar.

We all learned how to bake cakes and cookies ... with a lot of sugar ... and food coloring (chemical dyes). We ate fairly well in the summer with food from the garden and in the winter we ate what we canned in the fall. The canning process, of course, ... uses a lot of sugar ... and it's all cooked.

The bottom line here is that we ate a lot of what today I would call absolute junk. Consequently, at age 9, I developed an infection in my appendix and had to have surgery. (I explain in Volume II of this book series how and why appendicitis happens).

At age 13, just as I was getting ready to start high school, I experienced a rather severe "flu" that led to an ear infection that progressed to become mastoiditis. The entire mastoid bone behind my left ear had turned to mush and had to be removed.

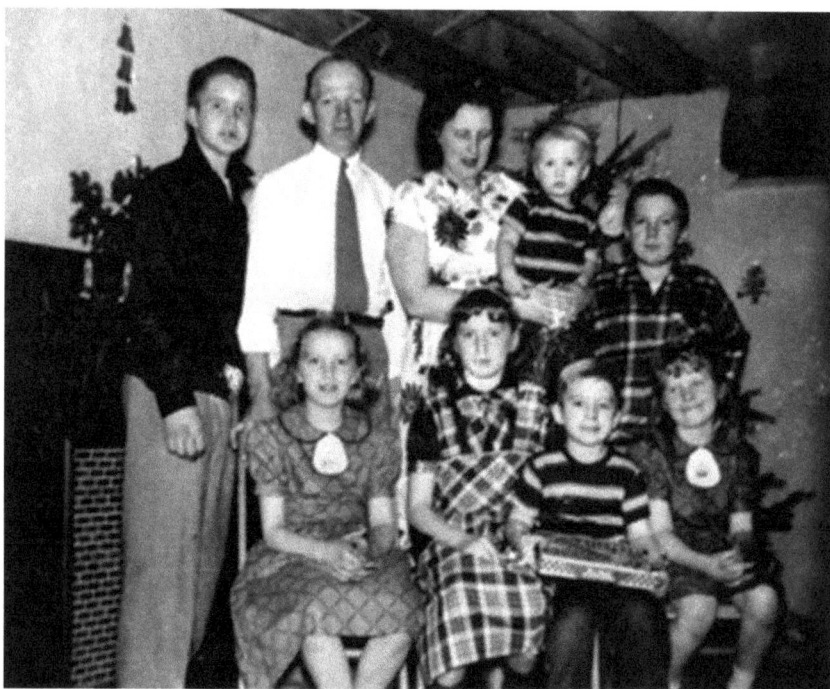

Me in 1953 (far left) two years after surgery

During the surgery to remove the infected mastoid bone, the surgeon accidentally severed my trigeminal nerve. This infection happened before antibiotics were used for every malady imaginable as they are today.

When I woke up after the surgery, I couldn't move or feel my face on the left side at all. They went back in to repair the nerve by splicing a piece of nerve from my neck into the damaged area.

PHIL SELINSKY, N.D.

It took a little over two years before I could eat or drink anything without having to hold my lips together with my fingers. I had to lie on my left side so that the pillow would hold my eye shut so that I could go to sleep at night.

On a humorous note, I told the girls that I had to kiss them twice because I could only give half a kiss at a time.

I know that other people have much more severe situations to endure in their life, but at the time, for me, this was an emotionally devastating experience.

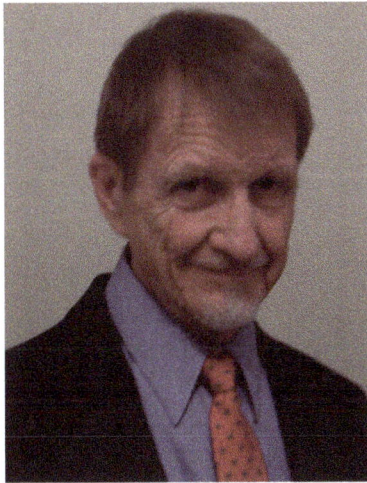

I was about 17 before I could feel anything on the left side of my face at all. It was totally numb for quite a while. Now, sixty years after the surgery, I have about 95% sensation back and maybe 60% muscle control and maybe 70% of the hearing in my left ear.

But I still can't whistle. That was the one thing that I missed most when it happened. I was a fairly good whistler before the surgery. Oh well. And oh yeah … now I can almost fake a full kiss. Yeehah.

From my teens to my late twenties, I had severe acne all over my body. Huge pustules would erupt on my face and back and chest. Many times the pustules would break open and soak through my shirt. That was rather embarrassing.

I had blinding migraine headaches almost every day. I had chronic low backaches. I frequently felt nauseous in the morning until I got going. I needed 10 to 12 hours of sleep every night. I had horrible body odor. My breath stank. My feet stank. I couldn't take off my shoes in a room without everyone running for the windows.

I frequently experienced hives (raised red itchy patches all over my body, especially on my chest if I leaned against something.

And of course, almost every tooth in my head was filled with mercury laden "silver amalgam" fillings, ... which probably explains my bizarre behavior now as well as throughout my whole adult life. Mercury is a toxic heavy metal that does in fact short-circuit brain cells and is a strong contributing factor to Alzheimer's, short term memory loss, and Parkinson's syndrome.

The good part is that all those experiences got me to where I am today, along with the knowledge and insight into my own as well as other people's behaviors and reactions.

By the way ... today at 73 years old, I need only 4 ½ to 5 ½ hours of sleep per night. I have no more acne or hives. I poop 2 – 3 times per day.

I have enough energy to consistently work 12 to 14 hours a day – 6 days. On Sunday I sleep in (6 hours) and in addition to normal household catch-up stuff, I make time to write this book.

Now when I hear people tell me "I can't do this or that because ...(fill in the blanks), I can say that I've been there and done that, and I know that you can do it because I've done it. You just need enough motivation.

I know most of the feelings and cravings that people experience in life because I have experienced the same feelings and cravings myself and have found out how to get on top of it all.

If the "machinery" of our digestive system is either **structurally** and/or **functionally** damaged or non operational, we will not be able to break the food down into small enough pieces to get into the blood to be able to build and/or repair worn out body parts. In addition, the rotting refuse that collects in the tissues of the body resulting from incomplete digestion is the direct cause of muscle and joint aches and pains. See the list below on page 13. WE EAT OUR PAIN.

The ultimate result of this structural and/or functional damage is "degeneration", which we recognize, over time, as emotional and physical aches and pains.

This condition frequently manifests in the body as:

Stress	Fibromyalgia
Indigestion	Muscle Cramps
Gas	Sciatic Pains--
Bloating	Irritable Bowel
Heart Burn (Reflux)	Celiac
Heart Palpitations	Leaky Gut
Mood Swings	Systemic Candida
Restricted Breathing	Chronic Bladder Infections
Bad Breath	Vaginal Yeast Infections
Depression	Prostate Inflammation
Painful Joints	Tumors and Growths
	… And many more.

My attempt with this book series is to show that this "**Human Machine**" that we drive around in for a time here on this planet is designed to "run" relatively trouble free. It's designed to adjust itself to its environment and to fix itself if and when it gets damaged along the way … if we don't sabotage it first, that is.

I have to emphasize here that the body is *designed* to do all these maneuvers. But if some of the parts become distorted or damaged along the way, or if the fuel supply is inadequate or tainted, this **Human Machine** will be thrown out of tolerance range, or "**ease of function**" and a state of "**dis – ease**" will ensue with its corresponding "check engine light" symptom profiles (See above list).

Western allopathic medicine has redefined the term, "**dis – ease**". Instead of a "*condition*" of dis – ease that can be changed with behavior and/or nutrition, we now refer to an "*entity*" called "**disease**" that we possess, and must attack with drugs and surgery.

This book (**Volume III**) will talk more about the **structural distortions** in the digestive mechanism itself, specifically the stomach, that can result in malfunction symptoms (aches and pains), rather than the discomforts caused by the disturbances in the **functional** aspect of the chemistry of the fuel supply (malnutrition) that I discuss in **Volume II**.

Hiatal Hernia Syndrome

It is an established biological fact that every life form must:

- ingest,
- digest,
- assimilate,
- excrete,
- be sensitive to its environment,
- be able to reproduce.

Any entity that can do all that is said to be "alive". If any one of these functions is distorted or disturbed or curtailed, the organism in question can no longer support life and will die. This is, of course, assuming a "natural" habitat.

"Survival of the Fittest" is a Universal Law that keeps all life forms in balance. The strongest of a species will pass on strong survival genes to the next generation. Weak life forms will die off and provide food for other life forms. That's the "natural" way!

In an "unnatural" habitat such as human beings have created for themselves, life can continue for a while, at some price in the form of inconvenience and/or discomfort and pain.

But eventually, the artificial life support system will fail and the organism in question will break down and cease to function.

Variations Of Hiatal (Hiatus) Hernia

This book will focus on the many variations of a condition called **"Hiatal Hernia"**. In this situation, the stomach, esophagus, and diaphragm are involved in an organ-damage condition that results in disturbed digestion with resulting blood pollution, which eventually can manifest as any number of degenerative conditions upon which Western Medicine has put an infinite number of labels. (See page 13 above for a partial list of symptoms related to a damaged digestive system.)

I have been studying this phenomenon for upwards of 40 years. My research has shown that this condition is responsible for a great many seemingly unrelated maladies or disturbances in the normal function of the human body including the recent apparent epidemic of diabetes, heart disease and cancer.

When I first started to pay attention to this phenomenon, I observed that close to 75% of all people that have come to me with a digestive problem, have shown symptoms of a **hiatal hernia** condition. As time goes on, and I become more familiar with all the symptom profiles, that percentage now stands somewhere closer to 95% to 98%.

I have been able to recognize seemingly unrelated aches and pains and organ malfunction as downstream effects of various forms of <u>hiatal hernia</u>.

There does not seem to be an age barrier to this condition. I have seen folks as old as 103 and babies just hours old displaying the undeniable symptom profiles.

In this book, I would like to present the physics, physiology, and chemistry that are related to creating this condition. In addition, I have discovered reliable behaviors and practices that will almost always relieve the agonizing pain and discomfort and misery that this condition creates in people's lives.

But the most important issue here is to learn how to prevent and control the problem <u>before</u> it develops.

As stated in all three Volumes of my book, **"THE HUMAN MACHINE ... A Trouble Shooter's Manual"**, repeated reference to the following concepts and principles is purposeful. My goal is to increase the likelihood that the reader understands that the violation of any of these principles listed here WILL result in some form of pain or discomfort or degeneration over time and that we humans have choices for behavior that can reduce or eliminate most pain. These concepts apply not only to the physical body, but also to the emotional body, the family body and the collective societal body.

- The Universe is always in balance. Balance = Homeostasis = Health
- "Symptoms of dis - ease" are the Universe in the process of returning to balance.
- Structure governs function ... the shape of something determines if or how it can be used.
- Environmental conditioning can bias a behavior <u>only</u> within its potential or structural capacity.
- Blood chemistry drives behavior and can and will trump or override intellectual choice.
- There is no mystery or magic ... just lack of information and understanding.
- Vibration is a physically expressive manifestation of Energy.
- The vibration of a medium creates shape in that medium.
- There is no free lunch ... Everything and every action consumes or changes energy (has a price).
- Survival of the fittest ... only the strongest and most resilient creatures survive to propagate the species (in a "natural" habitat, that is).
- Our greatest asset (the ability to adapt/accommodate) is also our greatest detriment. (The ability to change sometimes saves us from destruction in the moment. But then, continuous change sometimes places us too far from balance, which spells "destruction".)
- To be in integrity you must **live what you believe and believe what you live**. (Lack of "integrity" creates caustic stress, which is the ultimate killer ... not only of the body, but most importantly, of the character.

PART II

THE MECHANISM & SYMPTOMS

What I've Learned

Every life form eats something. Every life form on this planet has some mechanism or method to bring food from the environment into itself to provide materials for life maintenance. Every life form has some structure to catabolize or break the food down from its original form into usable building blocks.

Every Human Machine has a digesting system that must be able to break enough food down into the proper building blocks to keep the Human Machine in good repair, as well as to provide enough fuel to run all the system functions.

In the above paragraphs, I have discussed the **dis – ease** conditions that I experienced in my life that resulted in <u>**functional**</u> **distortions** due to the horrible eating habits in my growing up years.

This book (**Volume III**) will discuss the many **dis – ease** conditions and aches and pains that frequently result from <u>**structural**</u> **distortions** in the mechanism of the digestive system. You are either born with a defective part, or you experience trauma or surgery to change the shape and/or function of an organ or structure resulting in <u>**dis**</u> **– ease** (lack of ease - lack of homeostasis - lack of balance).

But when the smoke clears, it's ultimately the bad food choices over generations that distort the genes that result in the <u>**structural abnormalities**</u> with which we now suffer.

I must mention here that genes in their blueprint or pattern capacity will control the development and operation of structure as long as we are in *instinct* mode.

Humans have the capacity to overcome instinctive behavior and create new patterns of function and behavior. You can blame your parents and grandparents for your genetic distortions only until you become an adult and realize that you have choices. Please refer to **Volume I** for a discussion on the difference between *instinct* and *volition* (conscious choice) as well as childhood's attitude of "me, mine, and gimme" as opposed to responsible adult decisions and behavior.

Digestion - Putrefaction

As explained in Volume II, in order to get nutrient material into the cells of the human body for growth and repair, we must first be able to "digest" the food that we eat.

This means that the food must be broken down into small enough pieces that will pass through the up-take holes in the small intestine to get into the blood. If we have damaged or defective digestive organs, this process of digestion will be distorted or impaired.

Digestion is a timed, sequenced, and controlled catabolic process of organic material resulting in products that are useable by the human body for growth, repair, and fuel.

Putrefaction (rotting) is a random, uncontrolled, chaotic catabolic process of organic material that results in material that is no longer useful to the human body for any function.

At this point, if traumatic damage or a genetic defect in the structure of the organs distorts the digestion process, food material cannot break down into small enough pieces to pass into the blood within proper time constraints.

Similarly, if the structure is intact but the function is disturbed, the food will probably spend too much time in a warm, dark, moist place without adequate chemical control and will begin the rotting process. This will render the food no longer suitable for constructive use in the human body.

Timing is critical in the digestion process.

If you doubt that food rots inside the body, I ask only that you smell anything that comes from the body. If it stinks or smells peculiar, it has started the rotting process. The body and anything that comes from it, including urine, feces, perspiration and the breath, **should not stink**. They should have an identifying odor, but they should not be offensive. You should be able to tell the difference between feces and strawberries, but the smell of feces should not drive you out of the room.

Rotting

If organic material stays in a warm, dark, moist place for a period of time it will rot or ferment. It's supposed to do that. This is Nature in the process of completing a cycle.

All life forms go through:

- The Birth cycle
- The Growth cycle
- The Maturation cycle
- The Reproduction cycle
- The Death cycle
- The Decay cycle

When Consciousness leaves the life form, the life form returns to simple earth elements to be used once again in the construction of another life form.

Rotting is a one-way street. There is no return to usefulness (in the human body) once the food material has putrefied. The human body is designed and built to _suspend_ the rotting process for a period of time sufficient to allow a controlled, sequenced, and timed digestion of food material to take place.

If the timing is disturbed and/or the mechanism is damaged or distorted for any reason, **indigestion** takes place with resulting putrefaction or rotting inside the body. This results in a _condition_ of **dis – ease,** or lack of ease, or lack of homeostasis.

Please read Volume II of this **"THE HUMAN MACHINE … A Trouble-Shooter's Manual"** series for a more in depth explanation of this process and the importance of timing related to the rotting of food in the digestive tract.

First Let's Define the Terms

A **hiatus** is a port or an opening. In this instance we are referring to the opening in the diaphragm that lets the esophagus through from the mouth to the stomach. The stomach is located in the left side of the abdominal cavity just below the diaphragm.

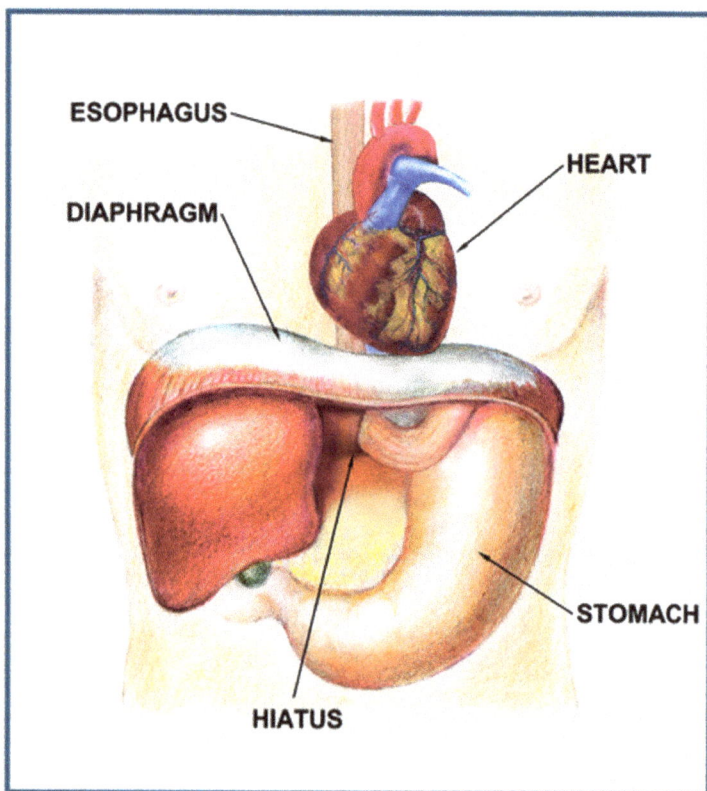

A **hernia** is a tear or a stretch. In medicine it is typically a tear or a stretch in muscle and/or connective tissue. Hernias can occur anywhere in the body. Common sites for hernias are the hiatus (opening) in the diaphragm, the umbilicus (belly button), lower abdominal hernia (muscle tissue separation just above the pubic hair line), and an inguinal hernia (fat and/or an intestinal strangulation into the inguinal canal). As we will discover further along in this text, all hernias are the result of a weak liver energy circuit.

In this case we are referring to the natural opening or **hiatus** in the diaphragm. The diaphragm is a parachute-shaped muscle that separates your chest cavity from your abdominal cavity. Your heart and lungs occupy space above the diaphragm, and your stomach and intestines live below the diaphragm.

Sometimes the muscles and connective tissue that form the hiatus or opening in the diaphragm become weak and then can easily stretch and / or tear. This **"hiatal hernia"** makes it possible for some of the stomach to possibly sneak up into the chest cavity through the stretched or torn hole or "hiatus" in the diaphragm.

This can put pressure on the heart resulting in heart palpitations and angina pains (pains under the shoulder blade and down the left arm). This phenomenon is many times mistaken for a heart attack and is treated with drugs and sometimes surgery that cause a myriad of down-stream side effects.

The stomach can also press against the lungs restricting breathing and causing pain and discomfort when breathing deeply. I have seen cases where Western medicine has surgically removed the first rib to reduce what they call "Thoracic Outlet Syndrome" … and I might add, to no avail. The problem is the stomach!!!! This actual invasion of the chest cavity by the stomach is an extreme condition and is relatively rare.

In the majority of cases that I have seen so far there may be *some* stretching or ballooning or slight aneurysm of the esophagus along with a slight herniation of the diaphragm. This condition causes an inflammation of the esophagus (esophagitis) that can result in a feeling like there's a pill stuck in the throat that just will not go down.

Considering the fact that the esophagus (the food tube) and the trachea (the wind pipe) join together just above the larynx (the voice box), the voice tone and quality may be affected. Singers, pay attention!!!

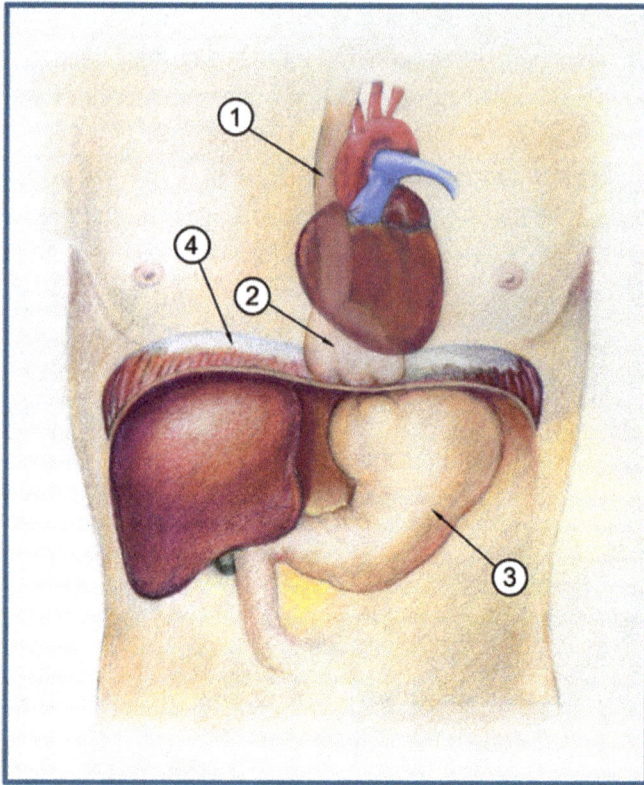

1) Esophagus
2) Part of the stomach (including the gastro-esophageal valve) in the "wrong place"
3) Stomach in the "right place" – where the stomach should be
4) Diaphragm

In addition, in light of the information in the ACHE AND PAIN chapter in Volume II, you may also sometimes feel pain along the side of the neck and at the top of the scapula in the upper back where the lavator scapulae muscle attaches. The pectoralis major muscles on the chest and the biceps muscles on the upper arms can also be sore and achy. Frequently the muscles along the side of the neck (sternocleidomastoid) will feel crampy and will limit the ability to turn the neck from side to side.

The muscles that control the attitude and position of the Atlas (the first cervicle vertebra) are affected by the stress on the stomach. Chronic

Atlas distortions (subluxations – a need to adjust or "crack" the neck) are blatant indications that the stomach is in trouble. Frequently the masseter muscle (chewing muscle) will be tight and will affect the TMJ (jaw joint).

There can also be a tightness and/or crampy sensation around the bottom of the rib cage (the attachment of the diaphragm). Soreness of the sternum (the breastbone) is common. This syndrome profile ranges from very slight naggy discomfort to severe pain and crippling dis - ease (lack of ease) symptoms.

If you've ever changed a baby boy's diaper, you may have noticed that when the baby is stressed as in preparing to poop or being exposed to cold, the scrotum shrivels and contracts up against the body. Similarly, when under constant emotional stress (adrenal overload), the stomach will sometimes shrivel and scrunch up against the diaphragm and cause all the symptoms that we have discussed here.

This is a survival reaction by the body. Like all living things, when presented with an actual or threatened danger, this machine was designed to revert to "instinctive" survival behavior, which is either "run like hell" or "stand and fight" or "freeze in position". (See Volume I for a discussion on "instinct".) In either situation, there is a need for 100% of available energy and resources to get you out of danger as quickly as possible.

The digestion system is one long muscular tube. Muscles use energy. The digestion system uses approximately 25% of the body's usable energy to digest food and move it through the tube from one end to the other. Therefore when the body senses "danger", it will shut the digestive system (the muscles of the intestines) down until you either slay the dragon or shinny up a tree, at which time digestion resumes.

However, the original design of this machine did not allow for the "danger" period to last all day and into next week. In our present day society, the periods of severe stress last a whole lot longer than they used to.

This means that food will be captured in a warm, dark, moist place for much longer than it would under normal peaceful conditions, resulting in putrefaction rather than digestion as explained earlier in this text. Specifically, the stomach will have a tendency to shrivel up against the diaphragm in what is described as a **functional** hiatal hernia as opposed to a **structural** hiatal hernia.

Probably the most frustrating issue with this **<u>functional</u>** hiatal hernia situation is that Western medicine will not be able to "see" anything wrong. The symptoms will be "sub-clinical". And yet you still feel all the pain and discomfort of a traumatized stomach, along with all the aches and pains and digestive disturbances described here in this text. You will then be labeled a hypochondriac and western medicine will order Valium or Prozac or Paxil or something equally as ridiculous.

When the stomach is stressed or traumatized, as in this situation with all the variations of the **hiatal hernia syndrome**, the stomach is physically injured. This means that it literally becomes inflamed and swollen. When it gets inflamed and swollen, there are two major situations that occur.

First, the stomach will be using more energy from the circuit in the attempt to heal the damage from the inflammation. Please refer to the chapter on "ACHES AND PAINS" in Volume II and "RESERVE TANKS OF ENERGY" on page 45 in this text to understand that the stomach will now draw extra energy from the muscles, resulting in pain and discomfort in the reflex areas related to the stomach.

Western medicine's protocol would be to prescribe Non- Steroidal-Anti-Inflammatory Drugs (N-SAIDS), which will cause more stomach damage leading to ulcers ... and they'll blame Helicobacter Pylori bacteria for the ulcers. (See next paragraph.)

The **second** and most important issue is that the stomach tissue now, because it is physically injured, cannot produce the digestive enzymes and acids in sufficient quality and quantity to properly digest your food (and protect you against H-Pylori infection). You now have organic material trapped in a warm, dark, moist place without the means to retard putrefaction. At this point you are a walking compost pile.

This means that you can be putting the best foods on the planet into your body ... you can literally live inside a health food store, and you will still experience putrefaction and fermentation in your stomach, which then manifests as gas and indigestion and bloating.

Remember, as stated earlier, that ANY organic material held in a warm, dark, moist place for a period of time WILL decompose – it will rot. The rotting food in your stomach will pass through the rest of your digestive system resulting in gas, cramping, inflammation, and serious malfunction and possibly eventual pathology (disease entities).

In addition, the 10th cranial nerve (Vagus Nerve) powers the entire digestive system complex, including the liver and the heart. When the stomach is injured due to surgery or constriction from the hernia, the Vagus Nerve will become irritated and possibly damaged. This nerve damage will affect all down-stream organs, structures, and processes. See "RESERVE TANKS OF ENERGY" on page 45.

This discussion would not be complete without mention of the latest weight loss fad ... the Lap Band and similar surgical interventions to limit the amount of food that can be eaten at any one time.

This whole book has focused on what happens when the stomach and/ or other digestive organs have been physically compromised. How much more damage can you do to your digestive process than literally surgically putting a "belt" around your stomach?

...Or by cutting some of the stomach out and attaching the small intestine to the esophagus?

When you interrupt the integrity of the vagus nerve (10th cranial nerve) with surgery, you will also influence all the other down-stream organs. I understand that sometimes there are situations where this type of surgery is required to save your life. In these cases the down-stream repercussions are understandable.

But I would strongly recommend that if you are contemplating this type of action as a weight loss maneuver, I have a better, cheaper, less permanent solution for you ... a six inch piece of duct tape placed strategically across that big gaping hole in the front of your face.

All that you would do with the Lap Band is restrict the volume of food that your stomach can hold. The duct tape would do the same thing quicker and less expensively. But seriously, in light of what we have discussed in these pages, look at the physical impairment and restriction that you place on the digesting process by intentionally injuring the stomach. Scar tissue impedes the flow of energy through the meridian channels (See page 39.).

Scar tissue and bruising as a result of the surgery WILL distort the energy flow through the stomach causing constant irritation of the stomach, which results in all the symptoms of the hiatal hernia.

The unfortunate folks who suffer from a physical hiatal hernia do not have a choice. They were born with the damage or the potential damage that develops over time. This book attempts to explain what can be done to live with that situation.

If you have a stomach that works, I would strongly urge you to keep it that way and try to limit the amount and quality of food volitionally. Food cravings are a blood chemistry imbalance, many times stimulated and triggered by an emotional stressor promulgated by a conflict between environment and structure (See Volume I.) Please refer to Volume II of this series for suggestions for weight control that do not involve surgery. The theme for the Volume II book is "Blood Chemistry Drives Behavior".

The primary job of the stomach is to suspend the rotting process until digestion can occur. **Remember that digestion is the timed, orderly, sequenced, and controlled break down of organic material**. The acid value in the stomach is of critical importance for this purpose. See page 75 in this text for a detailed explanation of the purpose and importance of HCl (Hydrochloric Acid) in the stomach.

Esphageal Aneurism

Another form of the **Hiatal Hernia Syndrome** is an **aneurism** of the esophagus. An **aneurism** is a ballooning or bulging of a tube such as the esophagus or a vein or an artery. An esophageal aneurism can develop as a result of continued reflux and/or a cramping or spasming of the gastro-esophageal valve.

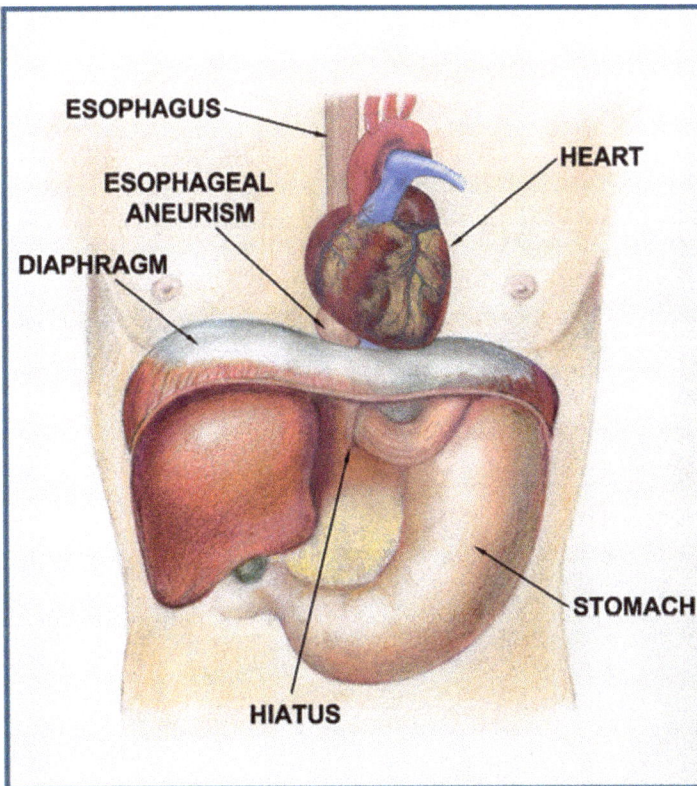

Food that is swallowed and cannot pass through the valve into the stomach can eventually cause a bulging or "hernia" or "aneurism" in the esophagus. This is a structurally weak spot in the muscle of the esophagus and can cause pain after swallowing and can result in a tear in the esophagus. This situation could be dangerous and potentially fatal.

NOTE: Any chronic and continued physical or chemical irritation of any tissue in the body can be a potential site for cancer to develop if other conditions are also met. (See this text page 84.)

Heart Burn ... Weak Les Valve

On the other side of the LES valve *spasm* conversation, resulting in the esophageal aneurism, is a *weak* LES valve, resulting in what western medicine calls Reflux Esophagitis.

The LES valve or the Lower Esophageal Sphincter opens and closes to let food from the esophagus into the stomach (a sphincter is a purse string or a pucker valve muscle, much like your mouth lips or your anus.).

As with the hiatus in the diaphragm, the strength and integrity of this muscle is controlled by liver energy. Therefore it is quite common to see both situations emerging simultaneously. But, keep in mind that they are two separate issues. One involves the hiatal hernia, which is a stretch or tear in the diaphragm, and the other is the lack of integrity of the LES valve between the stomach and the esophagus.

The hiatal hernia will result in pain just under the xyphoid process (that little dingy doo piece of cartilage hanging down just under the sternum or breast bone), plus possible heart palpitations, and sensations of something stuck in the throat, as well as feelings of shortness of breath.

The loose Lower Esophageal Sphincter will usually cause burning in the esophagus (heart burn). It is common to see both symptom profiles at the same time, but you can have one set of symptoms without the other.

If we're dealing with the hiatal hernia, it needs to be pulled down out of the hole to relieve the pain and discomfort. (See Part III page 112.) If the LES valve is left open, you will feel pain in the middle of your chest as the acid from the stomach sneaks up past the valve and literally burns the esophagus.

The stomach is protected from the hydrochloric acid with a layer of mucus, which the esophagus and the small intestine do not have. If we keep in mind that the original problem is the compromised liver energy, we can take a tablespoon of apple cider vinegar just before a meal, which should help to close the valve.

I have seen severe cases of loss of integrity of the LES valve where the apple cider vinegar does not close the valve. In these cases, it would be necessary to eat small meals and make sure the last meal is eaten a few hours before bedtime, to prevent the food from passing up through the valve while in a reclining position. It may be necessary to sleep on an incline with a wedge or pillows.

In extreme cases, western medicine has developed a mechanical spring device that can be surgically inserted over the esophagus to mechanically hold the valve shut until increase in the energy of the liver, enough to regain the strength of the LES valve, can be achieved. https://www.endtheweight.com/antireflux-gerd-surgery-norwalk.htm

THE PROCEDURE

The LINX system is a small surgical device which looks like a small bracelet. It consists of a flexible band of interlinked titanium beads with magnetic cores that create a ring shape. It has been designed to restore the body's natural barrier to reflux in those patients suffering from GERD (Gastroesophageal Reflux Disease). This LINX device is implanted around the esophageal sphincter. The normal sphincter is a circular band of muscle that closes the last few centimeters of the esophagus and prevents the backward flow of stomach contents. A weak sphincter allows acid and bile to reflux from the stomach into the esophagus. The purpose of the LINX System is to strengthen a weak sphincter using a minimally invasive laparoscopic technique. Strengthening the sphincter prevents the stomach's contents from backing up into the esophagus and creating reflux.

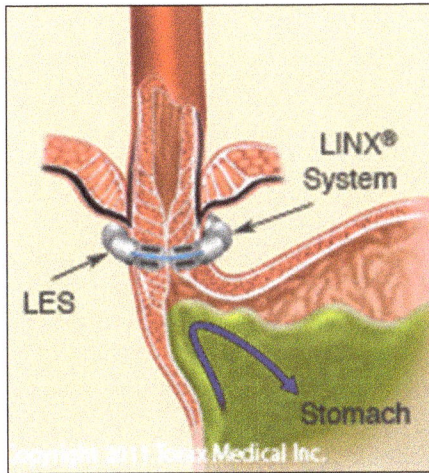

The LINX System is designed to help the LES resist opening to gastric pressures.

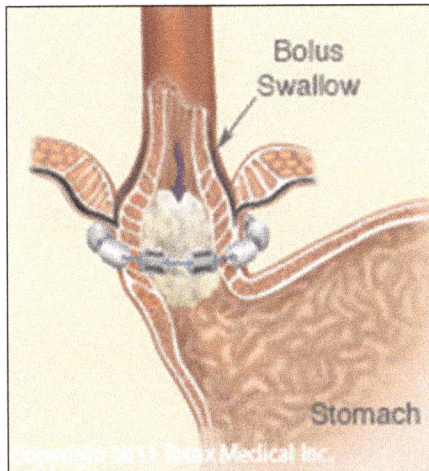

The LINX System is designed to expand to allow for normal swallowing.

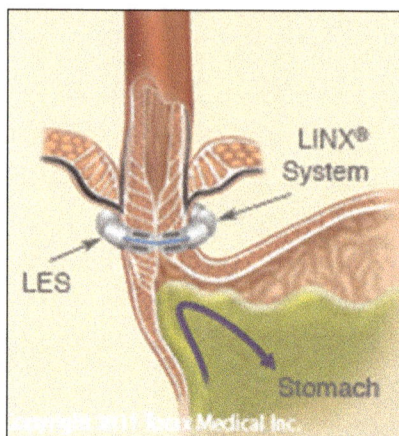

Magnetic attraction of the device is designed to close the LES immediately after swallowing.

When a person swallows, the magnetic force between the beads is overcome by the higher pressure of the force of swallowing. The device expands as the magnetic beads move apart on the titanium wires and allow the food and liquid to pass through it. After which, the magnetic beads return to their closed position and the valve closes. Because the magnetic beads open with pressure, the patient will be able to belch, vomit, and swallow normally. The LINX System eliminates the gas and bloating that is commonly associated with traditional reflux surgery.

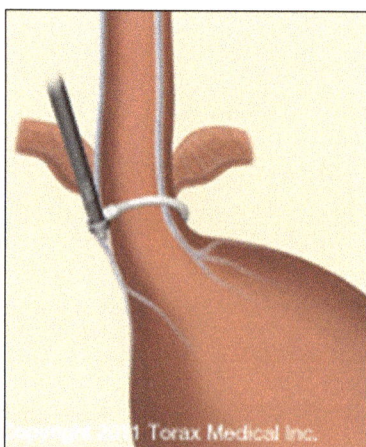

A precision sizing tool is used to determine the appropriate size LINX System.

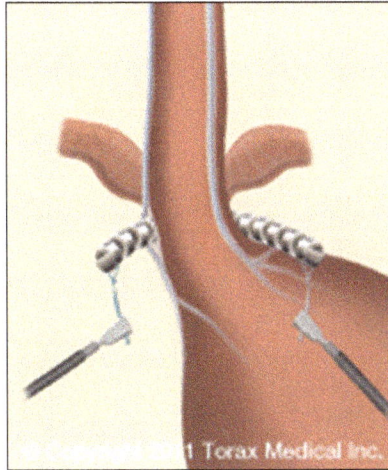

The LINX System is positioned around the LES using suture tails.

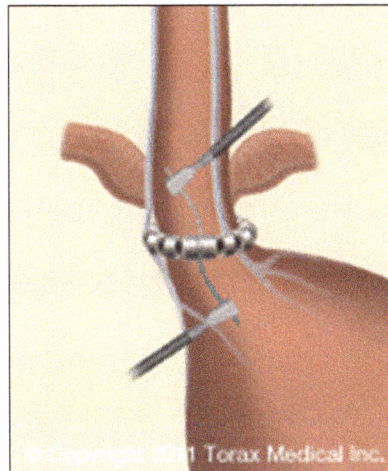

The ends of the LINX System are aligned and joined for suture closure.

LINX Reflux Management system has been designed for life-long use. The device is constructed of titanium, which has a long history in permanent medical implants.

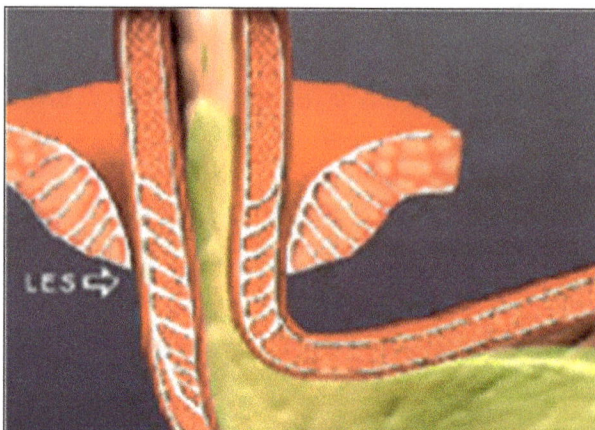

GERD results from a weak Esophageal Sphincter (LES). The weak LES allows acid and bile to reflux from the stomach into the esophagus.

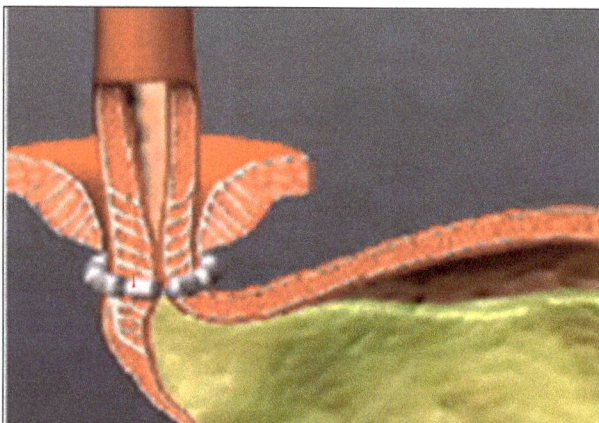

The LINX System is designed to augment the LES, with the aim of restoring the body's natural barrier to reflux.

Herniated Disc Problems

Most people in today's world have heard the term "herniated disc". This term refers to a tear or damage to the spacer, or wear-plate, in between the spinal vertebrae. As the spacer disintegrates due to dietary indiscretion, pressure is put on the nerves causing pain in the back and the legs.

This concept of dissolving bone and discs is covered in **Volume II of the HUMAN MACHINE BOOK**, but I would like to show here that both the "herniated" or damaged disc as well as the weakness or damage to the esophagus and/or diaphragm stem from the same root cause … blood chemistry and pH imbalance due to volitional dietary indiscretion and/or a structural defect such as a hiatal hernia.

Acid forming foods such as:

- Nicotine
- Caffeine
- Alcohol
- Refined sugar
- Refined flour
- Dairy products
- Drugs

tend to acidify the blood, which causes the body to pull calcium out of the bones to buffer the acid in the blood resulting in what western allopathic medicine calls *osteoporosis*. The blood must maintain 7.4 pH at all times, and therefore is constantly pulling calcium from the bones and depositing it into the blood stream to neutralize the acid in the blood caused from eating acid-forming foods listed above. The blood consequently then becomes supersaturated with calcium.

The calcium at this point will precipitate out of the blood and form deposits in arteries and joints and muscles resulting in aches and pains for which western allopathic medicine prescribes pain medication that further damages the stomach and overloads the liver. In addition, the deterioration of the spinal vertebrae shortens the height of the abdominal area and compresses the organs in the abdominal cavity, resulting in abdominal bulging and restricted intestinal and liver blood circulation and function.

This extra stress on the liver draws an excessive amount of energy from the liver circuit and has the tendency to put the body at greater risk for hernias, strains, sprains, and tears. (See the motor home example on page 52 and the free radical discussion on page 63 of this book.)

Examples of Disc Problems

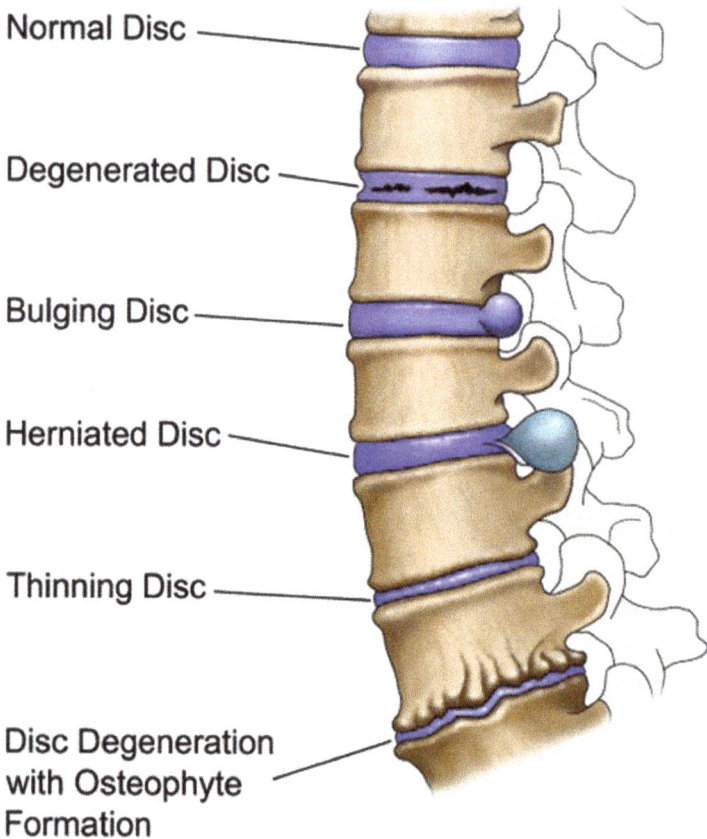

Normal Disc

Degenerated Disc

Bulging Disc

Herniated Disc

Thinning Disc

Disc Degeneration
with Osteophyte
Formation

Rivers of Energy

I must refer you back to Part V - ORGANS AND PRESSURE POINTS in Volume II of this **HUMAN MACHINE BOOK** for the background conversation for the existence of "rivers of energy" that drive each and every organ in the human body.

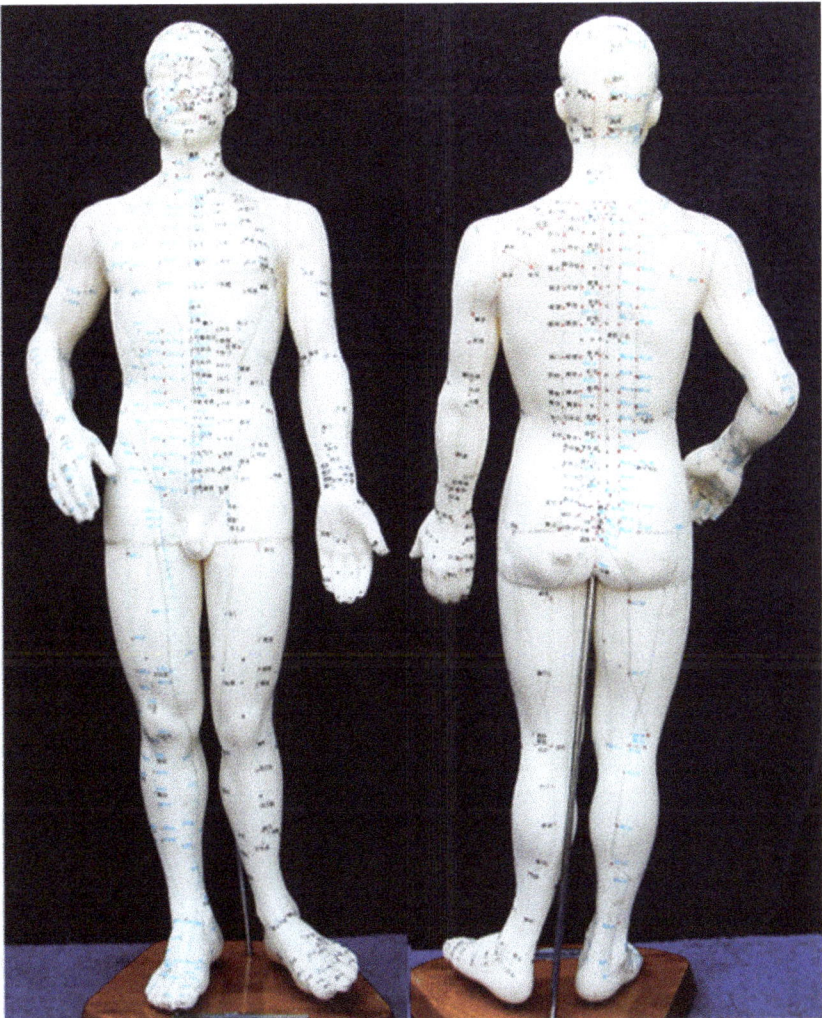

Every machine that is designed to "do" something must have an animating power source. Each of the organs in the human body has its own power circuit, much like the wiring in your house.

In your house, there are a number of electrical circuits that supply electrical power to different sections of your house.

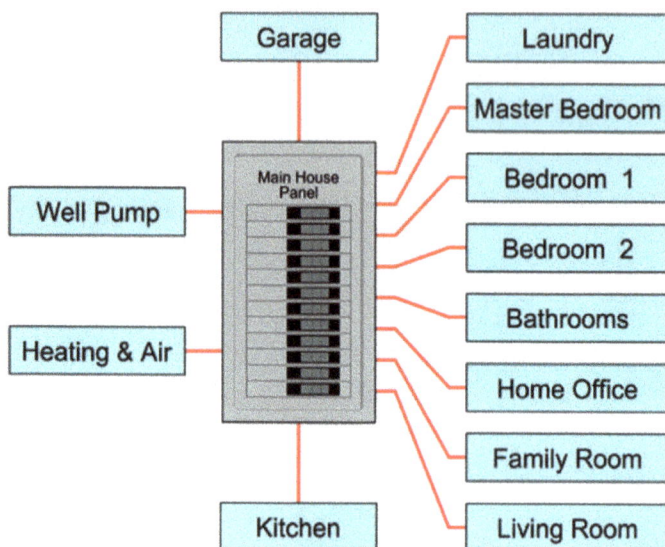

In your body, there are 10 electrical *"organ"* circuits and 2 electrical *"function"* circuits, making up a total of 12 major power circuits. There are minor circuits, but we will focus only on the major circuits here in this book.

Organ:	**YIN**	**YANG**
	Heart (He)	Small Intestine (SI)
	Spleen (Sp)	Stomach (St)
	Lung (Lu)	Large Intestine (LI)
	Kidney (Ki)	Urinary Bladder (Bl)
	Liver (Li)	Gall Bladder (GB)

Function: Circulation (Sc) or Pericardium (P) Triple Warmer (TW)

These "power" circuits in your body are different from the electrical wires in your house in that they are not hard physical wires that you can see with your physical eyes. These are electro-magnetic energy flows that follow actual physically determined pathways through the tissues of the body in a very specific direction. If the energy flows in the "proper" direction, the muscles that are "powered" by that circuit will be strong. If the energy flows in a reverse direction, the muscles will be weak and sometimes painful. (See pages 39 and 40.)

These "rivers of energy" can be detected by electronic devices and are influenced by electricity and magnetics even though they do not follow hard-wire pathways as do nerves.

Western medicine has a hard time with this phenomenon because unlike nerves that can be seen when dissecting a cadaver, energy meridians can no longer be detected after the death of the body.

It's also interesting to note at this point that the scientific community has documented a very slight weight loss at the time of "death". This infinitesimal loss of mass suggests that there truly is an "Energy Field" or Consciousness that actually disconnects from and leaves the physical body resulting in the loss of the animating electro-magnetic power. This loss of energy is commonly viewed as "death". Energy has mass and is influenced by gravity and therefore can be detectable in the physical dimension.

Each of these circuits supplies power to a different organ. Volume II covers all 12 circuits. We will only discuss the circuit that powers the liver here in this text.

We will *refer* to the other organs and their functions here, **but concentrating on and understanding the energy from the <u>liver</u> <u>circuit</u> is crucial to the development of the concept of the**

<u>Hiatal Hernia Syndrome</u> phenomenon.

Meridian Energy Flow Chart

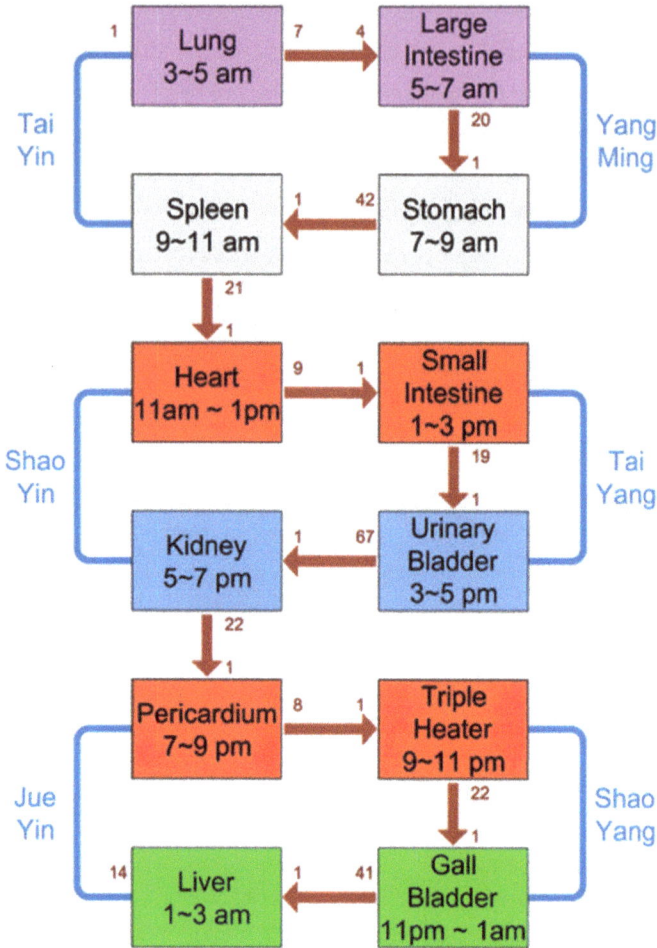

The arrows in this diagram show the sequence of the flow of energy through the system. The times listed here in the above chart show the orb of time that the particular meridian is "pulsing" with power. The "pulse" travels around through the whole system of 12 circuits every 24 hours. The "Schumann Resonance" or the electromagnetic pulse of the planet created by the spin of the planet Earth around its iron core and the interaction with the ionosphere results in nodal waves that appear in 2-hour cycles or pulses.

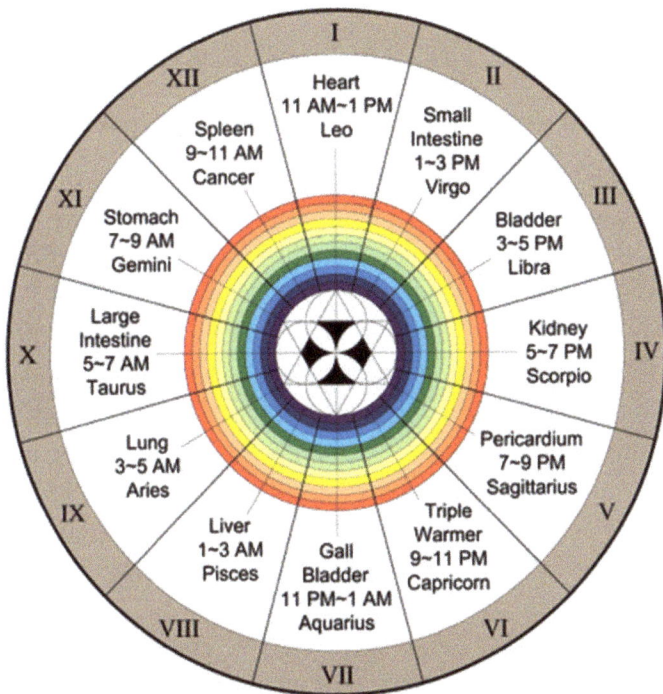

A circular graph would show that the "pulse" of energy flows from the Liver energy circuit back up to the Lung energy circuit. The Energy pulses through all the circuits every 24 hours. The times listed here on the chart are a period of 2-hour intervals for each meridian. They are local times (time of day where you are in the moment). The Chinese have translated the Schumann resonance pulse into a pictorial graph that shows how each organ in the body is individually energized every 24 hours. You could consider this process as "Cosmic Welfare". Everybody gets his/her "fair share".

If your "antennae" are up you will start to see that disturbing this natural pulse is the basis for jet lag. Local time pulses can get confused when traveling long distances. This confusion of energy in the circuits will affect the organs and correspondingly the related "surge/reserve tank" muscles as well as brain function. (See pages 45 & 46.)

Consciousness

In order to better understand the concept of the power that drives the organs, it is critical to first discuss the issue of Consciousness. You and I need to be on the same page here for us to proceed with the notion of "energy flow". I discuss this issue in more detail in Volumes I and II.

If you cannot entertain the thought of First Cause, or Prime Mover, or Infinite Intelligence, or Ultimate Engineer, or some other form of reference to a Higher Vibration Consciousness, this whole discussion will not make much sense to you. There is much evidence "out there" to support the fact that the physical body is "driven" by a Higher Vibration Consciousness.

Quantum physics is a branch of science that is now starting to recognize the existence of Consciousness. Some refer to it is as "The Field" or "The Matrix" or "Parallel Universe" or "The String Theory". Religions all throughout recorded history refer to the "soul" or the "aura" or the "spirit".

The Consciousness appears to have a plan. I'm not smart enough to tell you what Consciousness looks like, but I can certainly describe some of the apparent "mystical" phenomena that I see happening in the human body from an engineering perspective.

> *The laws of physics apply equally to all of the dimensions of Consciousness.*

Whoever put this thing (our body) together, wired each organ separately so that if one organ malfunctioned, the others could find a way to survive.

This "Ultimate Engineer" also saw the possibility of an individual organ needing to work "overtime" in case of an emergency survival situation and so "reserve tanks" were wired into the circuit.

> **Muscles** serve as "reserve tanks" or "energy capacitors" for the vital organs.

PHIL SELINSKY, N.D.

Reserve Tanks of Energy

THIS IS A _CRITICAL_ CONCEPT:

Muscles that serve as "reserve tanks" of energy for each of the vital organs are wired _in series_ with that specific organ. In a _series circuit_, the electricity flows through one device to another, eventually completing the circuit as opposed to a _parallel circuit_ in which each device is separately powered.

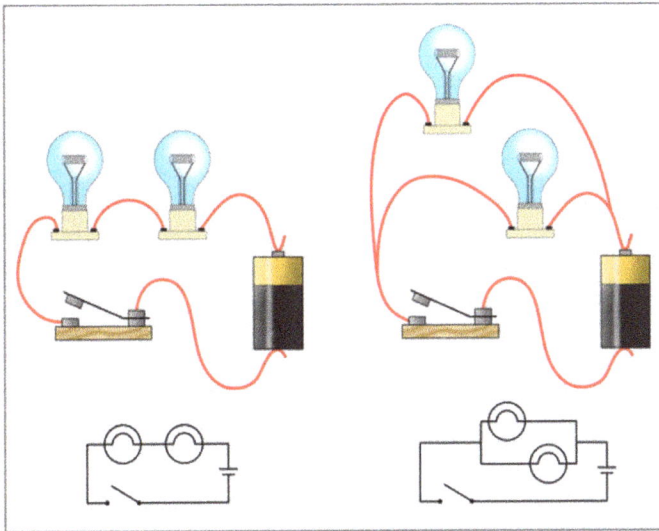

In a **series circuit** (left-hand side) the current flows through one globe after another, each being able to make use of only a part of the energy carried by the current. In a series circuit, if one of the globes blows and current can no longer pass through it, the current cannot flow in the circuit at all.

In a **parallel circuit** (right-hand side) the current can pass simultaneously through each globe and the energy of the current is available to each globe. In a parallel circuit, if one of the globes blows and current can no longer pass through it, the current can continue to flow through the rest of the circuit.

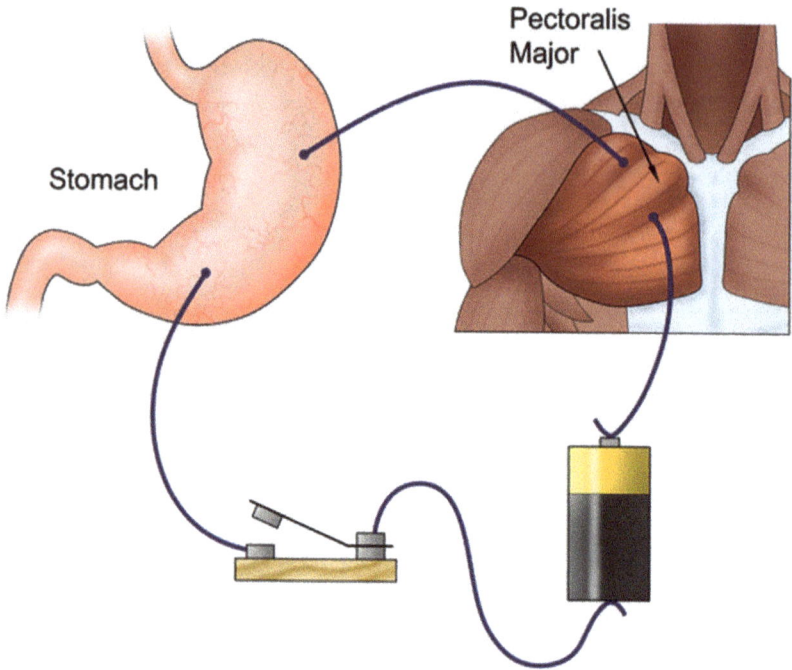

Muscles serve as "reserve tanks" of energy for each of the vital organs.

This way, we can test the strength and resilience of each muscle in the body to determine the "health" and vitality of the **vital organ** for which it serves as a reserve energy supply.

If the reserve tank is low in energy (weak muscle), we can assume that the **vital organ** that is wired in to this particular muscle is also low in energy, and is probably showing symptoms of malfunction. This picture (above) shows one of the muscles that are powered by the stomach energy circuit. Pain or weakness here would be an alarm bell signal or a "check engine light" for a stomach issue. If the stomach is irritated or impinged in some fashion, it will draw more energy to be able to survive. It may need to "work overtime" attempting to process a large meal or it may be attempting to repair itself from an injury such as a hiatlal hernia or an ulcer, in which case, it will draw energy from the muscle resulting in weakness and possible cramping and pain in the indicator muscle.

Muscle Testing Theory

We can now test the strength, resilience, and sensitivity of each muscle in the body to determine the "health" and vitality of the vital organ for which it serves as a "reserve energy" supply because the organ and the muscle *together* complete a circuit.

If a muscle tests "weak" and/or painful, it shows that the power to the "circuit" is low or restricted, resulting in low organ energy. This frequently manifests as symptoms of **dis – ease** in the organ function.

In addition to physical function, each **vital organ** has *energetic* duties throughout the body along with the functional responsibilities of that specific organ.

Under extreme conditions, the survival of the organism is the first order of business, so that when there is a threat to survival, the stressed organ is number one priority over muscles for all the available energy in the body.

This means that the energetic duties as well as the reserve supply muscles related to that particular organ will suffer a loss of functional capacity most often resulting in aches and pains, for which we take drugs, which cause more aches and pains. (See the Motor Home Model on page 52.)

For a video demonstration of muscle testing to determine the integrity of a circuit, see my web site www.thehumanmachine.com.

I must emphasize here that this muscle testing procedure has gained wide spread usage in recent months. Many people are using an "indicator muscle" which is an easily accessed muscle to test. Many people use either the deltoid or the pectoralis major clavicular in the arm to test for strength or weakness after asking a question or putting some substance in the body's magnetic field. This technique has been taught by the ICAK to doctors to be able to determine subtle and occult imbalances in the body's energy field and corresponding organ and muscle function.

Because it is easy to "influence" or to intimidate or suggest a response to the question based on what the tester would like to see, I prefer to stick to the "hard-wire" testing of different muscles that are directly related to the organ function that in turn relates to the presenting ache or pain or dysfunction. Some people are good at this "airy fairy" stuff, but I don't trust it. I'm still a skeptical engineer.

Liver Energy Meridian Flow

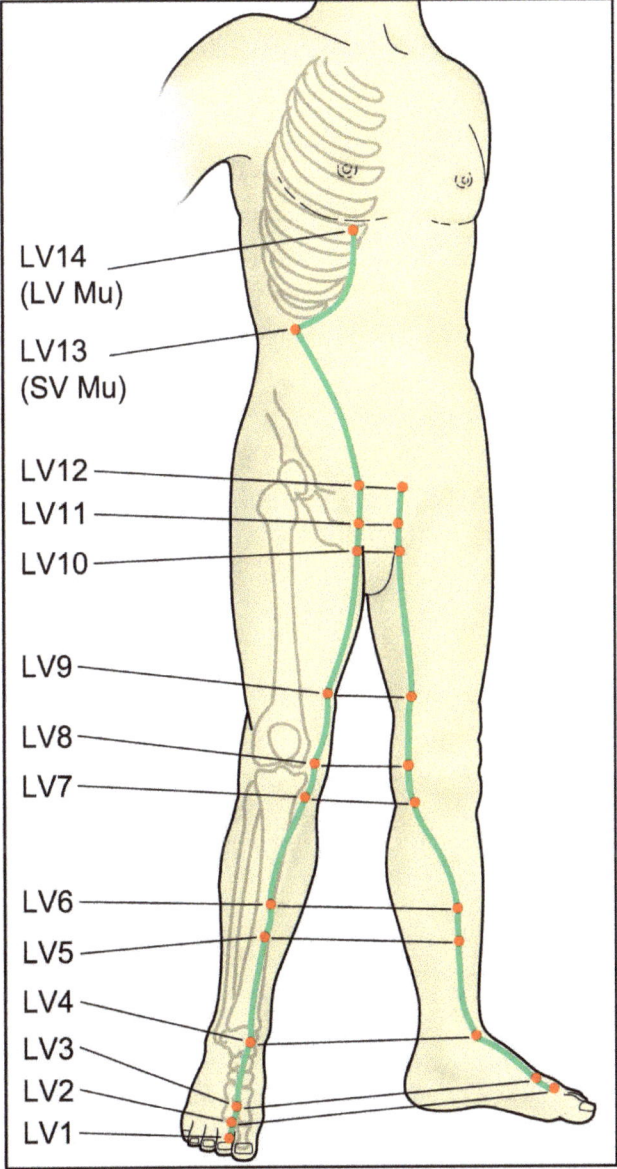

LV14
(LV Mu)

LV13
(SV Mu)

LV12
LV11
LV10

LV9

LV8

LV7

LV6

LV5

LV4

LV3

LV2

LV1

Liver Energy

In Chinese Medicine, the energy that drives the liver also is responsible for the integrity of muscle and connective tissue in the human body. In other words, the strength, resilience, flexibility, and tone of all muscle and connective tissue in the body are the responsibility of the liver energy. Please keep in mind that all the veins and arteries and the heart muscle itself, as well as all the digestive system muscles are all also affected by the integrity of the liver circuit.

This means that if the liver is compromised or encumbered in any way (as in taking drugs or processing pollutants from the large intestine), the liver energy is consumed in preserving the survivability of the organism at the expense of the peripheral muscle and connective tissue. The result here is that because of the energy deficit in the liver circuit, the muscles and connective tissue are placed at risk of damage from over use or undue stress. Fewer muscle cells are pulling the load for the whole muscle, which puts a strain on the working cells. (Kinda' reminds me of the way the U.S. economic system operates.) In addition, the loss of energy causes spasms, which results in pain and discomfort.

The more stress and strain that is placed on the liver, the less energy is available to support the integrity of muscle and connective tissue. This individual with low liver energy is now at greater risk for muscle tears, strains, sprains, hernias, and prolapses (sagging tissue), in addition to suffering digestive system dysfunction. Remember that the alimentary canal is one long muscular tube.

I refer you back to Volume I of the **HUMAN MACHINE BOOK** for the discussion on **structure/function**, and the reasoning behind how a genetically weak liver circuit can manifest as genetically weak connective tissue.

This results in weaker genes passed on to the offspring so that in generations down stream, babies are born with weak liver circuits and consequently at genetically greater risk for weak connective tissue integrity.

We see this manifesting today as an epidemic of **hiatal hernia profiles** with the corresponding plethora of digestive problems resulting in an unending list of **"degenerative dis - eases"**.

Motor Home Model

To illustrate this point, let's look for example, at a motor home. The gas tank supplies the engine with fuel so that the vehicle can move from one place to another. But the air conditioner and the compressor motor and the generator motor also draw gasoline from the same main tank.

When the gas gauge shows 1/4 tank, most modern motor homes are designed to shut off the generator or the air conditioner or the compressor to conserve enough fuel to get the vehicle to a gas station to refuel.

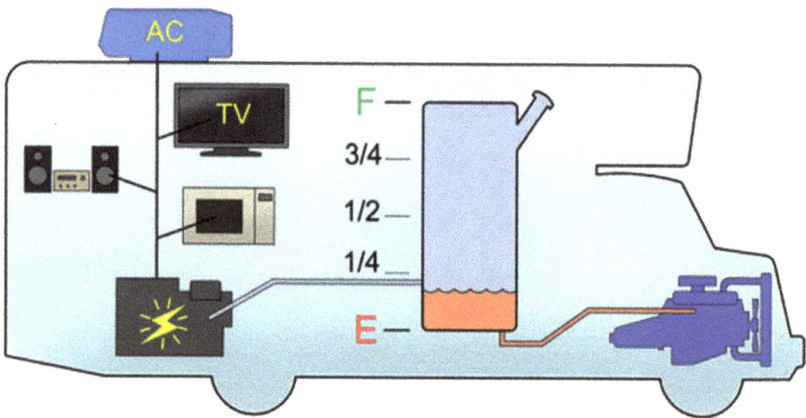

A similar energy or fuel supply condition exists in the human vehicle (body) with respect to organs and muscles. In the motor home, without the engine, the motor home is somewhat worthless for moving you down the highway. Consequently the engine has priority over all the other accessories when the fuel supply runs low.

In your body, without the organ, you die. So, similar to the engine in the motor home, the organ gets first dibs on the energy available in the "circuit".

When we experience "low liver energy", for example, the muscles that are on the same energy circuit are considered expendable by the body with respect to the liver, which is a <u>vital</u> <u>organ</u> and are "shut down" until more energy is available.

If you try to use the muscle that has been "shut down", you are at risk of physically damaging the muscle. Sprains, strains, torn muscles, and hernias are examples of attempting to "push" a muscle past its energy capacity in the moment.

Some people are born with hernias. Some people are born with a weakness that results in hernias later in life because they exacerbate the existing weakness by putting a further load on the liver by engaging in an indiscriminate life style. Please reread Volume II for foods that tax the liver system and good foods that benefit the body. Also see page 66 in this text for food combining suggestions.

> **I must emphasize once more that long-term chemical and energetic stress on the liver WILL eventually affect the heart negatively. <u>Heart</u> <u>attacks</u> <u>start</u> <u>with</u> <u>liver</u> <u>attacks</u>!!!**

5 – Element Theory

According to the **5-Element theory of Chinese medicine**, the "Sheng" cycle or the "Creation" cycle states that Fire creates Earth, which creates Metal, which creates Water, which creates Wood, which in turn once again creates Fire.

In the diagram below, notice the arrows pointing to a clockwise rotation. Each element "creates" the next in the clockwise direction.

The Fire element corresponds to the heart. The Wood element corresponds to the liver. If the Wood element does not furnish "fuel" for the Fire to burn, the heart energy diminishes. If the Wood energy remains weak over time, it will "put the Fire out". If the liver energy remains weak over time, the heart energy will suffer.

I say again, **Heart attacks start with liver attacks!!!**

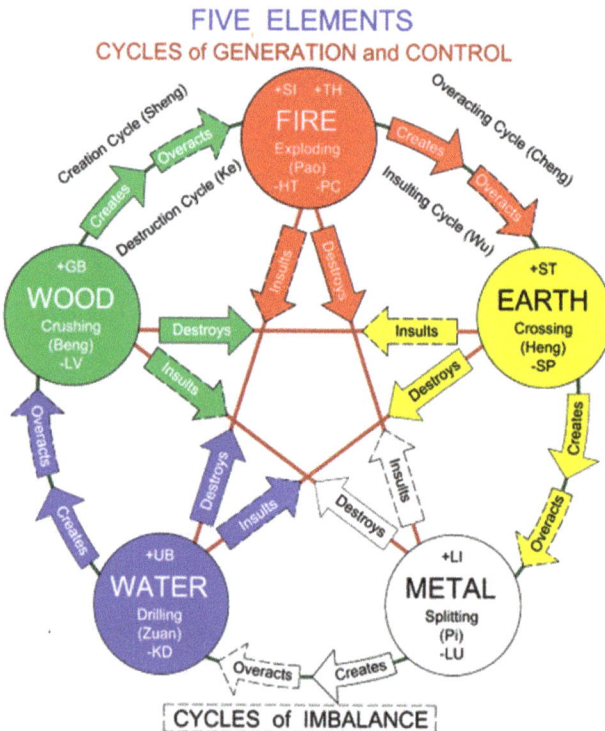

FIVE ELEMENTS
CYCLES of GENERATION and CONTROL

CYCLES of IMBALANCE

Let's go back to our motor home example. If you're traveling along a relative straight highway, the fuel consumption will be somewhat constant and predictable and you can be running the generator and air conditioner while cruising down the highway. But if you travel a long distance between fuel stops and you run low on fuel or if you happen to be in a rather mountainous area, hauling a heavy motor home up a steep grade for a long distance you're going to consume more fuel than you would on straight ground.

This means that if you start getting low on fuel, the air conditioner and generator might be shut down temporarily until you fill up the tank again.

If you have a small "gas tank" to begin with, you might not be able to run the "accessories" at your convenience all the time. You then might have to "ration" the use of the "accessories".

You could quite possibly have developed a "kink" in the fuel line somewhere so that you cannot get enough fuel to travel as fast as you would like. Or your "tank" might be clogged up with "rust" or "debris" and cannot hold a "full tank of fuel", which would limit the distance that you could travel and the number of accessories that you could use at the same time.

If the liver is clogged up with chemical debris from an indiscriminate lifestyle, it may not have enough energy available to "run" all the accessories (muscles) at the same time and may have to shut some of them down in order to keep the "machine" running (stay alive).

Remember that the main driving force of all life forms on this planet is <u>SURVIVAL</u>. The organism will sacrifice non-essential structures and activities in order to <u>survive</u>.

This automatic temporary shutdown phenomenon will many times result in chronic aches and pains in the areas listed below due to the low overall liver energy. If a business does not take in enough profits to make payroll, some of the workers will not get paid. The unpaid workers will stop working. Because non-essential activities like building maintenance, internal transportation, and quality control are cut, production slows down. The workspace clogs up. Trash builds up. Sanitation becomes a problem. Communication breaks down. Machinery starts to wear out because of lack of maintenance and spare parts.

The **HUMAN MACHINE** is a factory. It's a business. Like any other business, it must be maintained adequately in order to function harmoniously. (The following list of liver energy shutdown symptoms is "borrowed" from Volume II of **THE HUMAN MACHINE ... a Trouble Shooter's Manual.**)

Common Liver Overload Symptoms

Some common symptoms related to liver overload are:

- pain in the temples,
- pain between the shoulder blades,
- pain on the inner thigh just above (proximal to) the knee joint,
- chronic ear infections,
- nausea,
- loss of balance,
- hepatitis (inflammation of the liver),
- muscle aches and pains (fibromyalgia),
- sagging organs (prolapse),
- tearing or stretched connective tissue (hernia),
- sagging skin (old age),
- dry scaly skin,
- skin discolorations (old age spots or "liver spots"),
- behavior stemming from or about anger and/or rage

If these conditions persist over time, you can expect a heart problem to appear (See page 54 for 5-Element explanation).

> *Parents distort their liver genes by exposing their bodies to chemicals and toxins that stress the liver. Over a number of generations of liver insult, the successive parents pass on weaker and weaker genes to their offspring so that eventually the present generation is born with compromised immune systems and liver and pancreas capacities. This leads to potentially weak muscle and connective tissue, which leads to increased risk for hernias.*

We'll discuss further along in this text how and why an indiscriminate life style could or would impact the ability of the liver to function properly. Every part and piece of our bodies has a specific job and/or function. There is a reason that everything <u>exists</u> and <u>does what it does</u>.

> *Second-guessing and disturbing what Nature does is a dangerous practice.*

pH (Potential Hydrogen)

The human digestive system is designed to provide a supportive environment for the proper digestion of food material. Most of us have heard the term "pH". Potential Hydrogen or pH is a method of grading or measuring the acid/base condition of the local environment. Let me digress for a moment to explain what acid/base is.

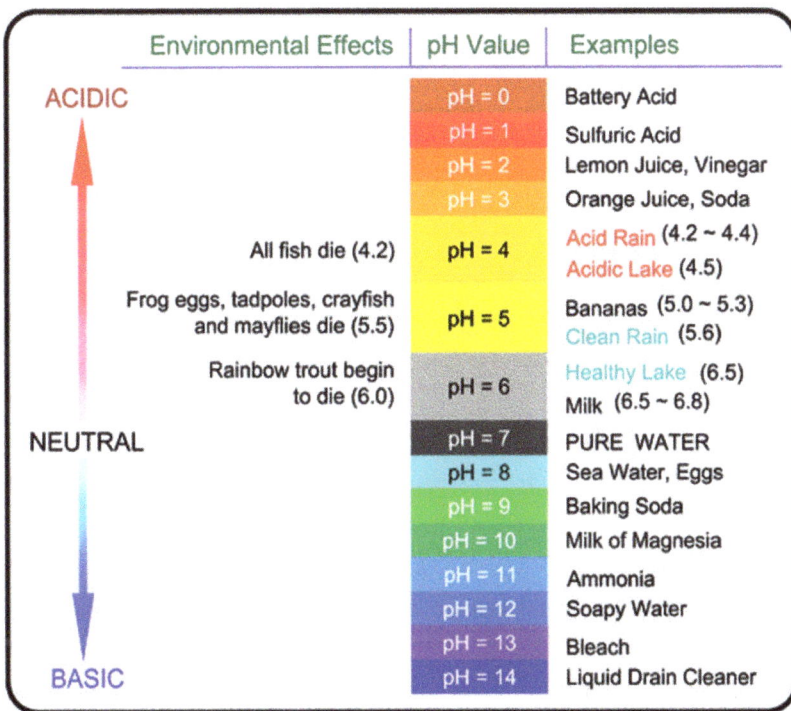

	Environmental Effects	pH Value	Examples
ACIDIC		pH = 0	Battery Acid
		pH = 1	Sulfuric Acid
		pH = 2	Lemon Juice, Vinegar
		pH = 3	Orange Juice, Soda
	All fish die (4.2)	pH = 4	Acid Rain (4.2 ~ 4.4) Acidic Lake (4.5)
	Frog eggs, tadpoles, crayfish and mayflies die (5.5)	pH = 5	Bananas (5.0 ~ 5.3) Clean Rain (5.6)
	Rainbow trout begin to die (6.0)	pH = 6	Healthy Lake (6.5) Milk (6.5 ~ 6.8)
NEUTRAL		pH = 7	PURE WATER
		pH = 8	Sea Water, Eggs
		pH = 9	Baking Soda
		pH = 10	Milk of Magnesia
		pH = 11	Ammonia
		pH = 12	Soapy Water
		pH = 13	Bleach
BASIC		pH = 14	Liquid Drain Cleaner

In traditional chemistry, "elements" are composed of "atoms", which are in turn composed of "protons" and "electrons". According to quantum physics, these subatomic particles are observed to be nothing but waveforms, but we will keep this discussion of molecules limited to the mundane (low level) physics of the proton and electron behavior here in this text.

Atom Identity vs Electrical Charge

The number of ***protons*** in an atom determines the **identity** of the element.

The number of ***electrons*** in an atom determines the **electrical charge** of the atom.

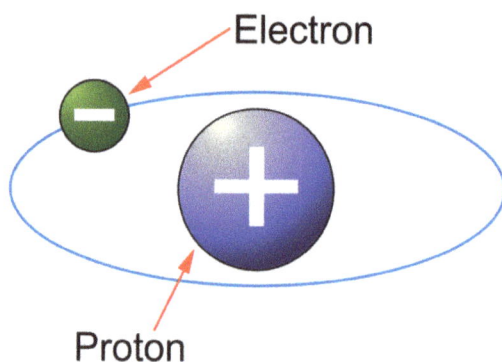

| 1 H | | | | 5 B | 6 C | 7 N | 8 O | 9 F | 2 He |

Protons have a positive electrical charge. That means that for every proton in an atom there must be one negatively charged electron to keep the atom electrically balanced. Adding more electrons to an atom only changes the **electrical charge**. *It does not change the identity of the atom.* The identity of an element is changed by adding protons. See the partial periodic table above.

One proton with one electron creates the element Hydrogen. If the electron is removed from a neutral Hydrogen atom (one proton plus one electron), we still have Hydrogen with a positive charge.

A hydrogen atom with a positive electrical charge is considered <u>acidic</u>.

If an extra electron is added to a neutral (one proton plus one electron) Hydrogen atom, a negatively charged Hydrogen atom will result.

A Hydrogen atom with a negative electrical charge is considered basic or <u>alkaline</u>.

An acid will be attracted to or will steal electrons from another molecule or compound, changing the shape and configuration of the affected molecule. This can change the function of the molecule (See Volume I – Structure/Function for a discussion on how shape governs function. You can also get a "taste" of the concept if you go to my web site <thehumanmachine.com> and click on BOOKS Volume I - "STRUCTURE/FUNCTION").

An alkaline or base will donate electrons to a molecule or compound, again, changing the shape of both structures. Sometimes two molecules will "share" one electron thereby creating a new structure.

This acid/base phenomenon is utilized very efficiently in the digestive system. Some foods need an acid environment to break down properly and some foods need an alkaline (base) environment to proceed through the digesting process.

Some foods will break down if an electron is "<u>stolen</u>" from the molecule resulting in the food molecule becoming unstable.

This action results in the <u>controlled</u> <u>catabolic</u> process called "*<u>digestion</u>* in an *<u>acid</u>* environment".

I mentioned in the first part of this book that the *Universe is always in balance*. Remember that acids are atoms or compounds that are missing electrons. To balance themselves they will "pull" an electron from any nearby available substance. An acid environment will "steal" electrons from the food molecule in question.

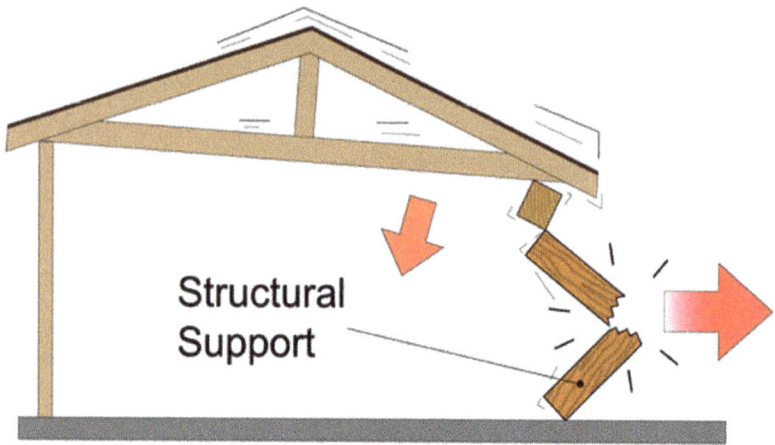

Structural Support

It's like pulling the pin on a hand grenade or removing a support beam from a building. It will blow up or fall apart. The body can now get the "pieces" into the blood for construction and repair of body parts.

Free Radicals / Antioxidants

Parenthetically, this is the same concept or argument that is made when discussing **"free radicals"** and **"antioxidants"**. These are "fad" words used to explain the process of "rusting" in the body. When electrons are attracted away from a substance, the substance rusts or decomposes. When body parts rust or decompose because of "free radicals" in the blood, tissues or organs become distorted and/or non-functional.

This process advances the aging phenomenon. Rusting in the digestive tract (digesting) is a good thing. Rusting in the tissues outside of the digestive tract is NOT a good thing.

Electrons are the "currency" of the cellular economy.

No electrons → depression – destruction. Electrons – a – plenty → booming cellular economy. See Volume II for further discussion. Also see "Electrical Nutrition" and "Asea" on my web site under LEARNING CENTER.

Some foods will break down when an electron is "acquired". An alkaline environment is necessary to supply extra electrons so that the food molecule can break down or digest. This is like driving a wedge into a structure to break it apart.

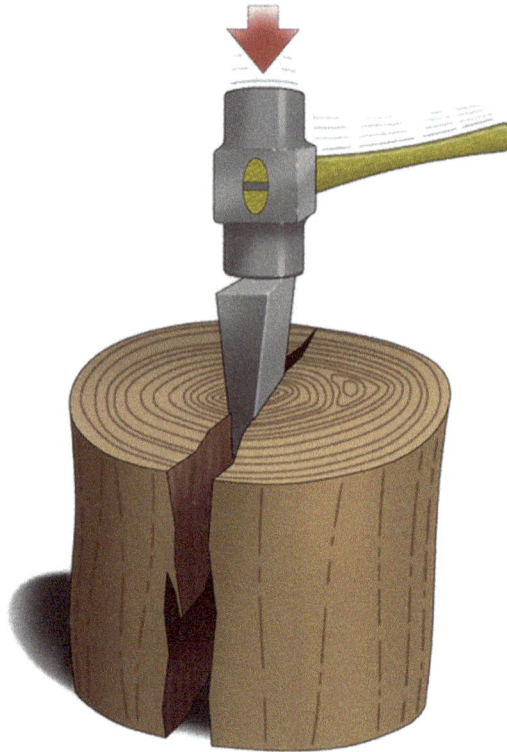

This action results in the <u>controlled</u> <u>catabolic</u> process called "_digestion_ in an _alkaline_ environment".

The pieces, once again, can be used for body growth and repair. Failure of the process (failure to digest properly) at this level will result in ultimate starvation. Actually, a more apt term would be "selective starvation". The body may have adequate nutrients for a number of parts and activities, but not for certain critical functions. This condition will result in a state of **dis – ease or de – generation or aging.**

PHIL SELINSKY, N.D.

Controlled Environments

It should now be obvious that an acid environment cannot supply "wedges" to foods that need extra electrons (wedges) to break them down.

There is an <u>absence</u> of "wedges" (electrons) in an **acid** environment. Food molecules that break down when electrons are "stolen" need an acid environment to break down.

An **alkaline** environment has an oversupply of electrons and therefore cannot attract electrons away from the food molecules that need to lose electrons in order to break it down properly. *We need to be clear on this subject.*

Remember that time is a critical function in the digestion process. If there are too many electrons available to a food requiring an acid environment (no electrons), digestion timing may be affected, resulting in putrefaction. Similarly, if there are not enough electrons available to a food that needs an alkaline environment (many electrons) to break down adequately, time may also run out for this food resulting in putrefaction.

If too much time elapses in a warm, dark, moist place, without the proper controls, putrefaction will occur instead of digestion. If the "timer" goes off before the "job" is done, fewer nutrients are available and more contaminants will overload the system, requiring more energy for clean-up and less for desired activities.

In a healthy human, the mouth should be alkaline, the stomach needs to be acid, the small intestine must be slightly alkaline, and the large intestine requires a weak acid bias. If these conditions are disturbed or altered for any length of time, a state of **dis – ease** results.

Food that DOES NOT break down, or catabolize adequately, cannot be used by the human body for the purposes of building and repairing damaged or worn tissue.

Once again, organic material that is trapped in a warm dark moist place for an extended period of time, without chemical intervention, will rot and become toxic to the human body.

Food Combining Suggestions

Rule #1: Drink pure chemically uncontaminated mineral rich water.

REASON: The body needs water to digest protein and to flush waste material from the tissues. A water molecule is required for breaking a protein molecule into separate amino acids for cell construction and repair.

Rule #2: Eat fruit by itself. Do not put fruit in the stomach with anything else.

REASON: Fruit is already mostly sugar. It needs very little further digestion. It needs to leave the stomach as soon as possible to avoid fermentation in a warm, dark, moist place (the stomach).

Sugar -> alcohol -> formaldehyde (embalming fluid).

Rule #3: Do not mix starches and proteins in the stomach at the same time.

REASON: Starches require an alkaline digestive environment and proteins require an acid environment for digestion. Acids and alkalines neutralize each other resulting in putrefaction instead of digestion. See discussion on Controlled Environments above.

Rule #4: Do not mix concentrated foods in the stomach at the same time. (See list below)

REASON: Concentrated, complex foods require a digestion sequence ranging from acid to alkaline. The priority and sequencing of digestion is different for each food group and therefore would result in indigestion if more than one sequence were combined and superimposed on each other. The timing for some acid components in one group would overlap the timing for some alkaline components in another group and would result in putrefaction. (See comparison chart on page 68.)

Concentrated (Complex) Foods

Group #1: Meats and anything produced with or from animals such as dairy, eggs, etc.

Group #2: Grains – rice – millet – oats – wheat – barley, etc.

Group #3: Legumes – Beans – dried peas, etc.

Group #4: Tubers – potatoes – peanuts, etc.

Rules for Complex Foods:

1) Choose one food from the above groups for the main dish for the meal.
2) Do not mix a representative of one group with a representative of another group. (Do not mix the groups together in the stomach at the same time.)
3) Eat the chosen main dish with a vegetable and/or a salad to make a meal.
   - Vegetables (including greens) digest relatively simply in a wide range of pH. Therefore they can safely be combined with any representative of the above 4 groups.
   - All foods are composed of proteins, carbohydrates, and fats in varying degrees of concentration. Most foods are predominantly one or the other. In the "concentrated" food groups, molecular bonding is more complex than simple fruits and greens. This requires a more complicated and sequenced breakdown process. Controlled acid/alkaline (pH) changes are necessary to break the complex molecular bonds in sequence so that "proper" and complete digestion occurs rather than partial digestion and some putrefaction. Putrefaction (rotting)

takes place when the breakdown process happens randomly (uncontrolled).

- The body scans the DNA of the food that has just been eaten and initiates the proper pH environment for that particular food to digest in proper sequence. This is an "energy field" process and falls in the realm of Quantum Physics. There is an energy field overlap that allows the resonant readout to take place, preparing the digestive system for the intended food consumption before the food actually touches the tongue. The body energetically "feels" the food.

The required pH environment and sequencing may be different for different concentrated foods. Too many sequencing messages from too many different complex foods at the same time causes the sensing computer to "lock up" resulting in random chaos.

Therefore, combining these "concentrated" foods in the stomach at the same time may cause a disruption in the pH sequencing, thereby resulting in random molecular bond breakdown (putrefaction by definition).

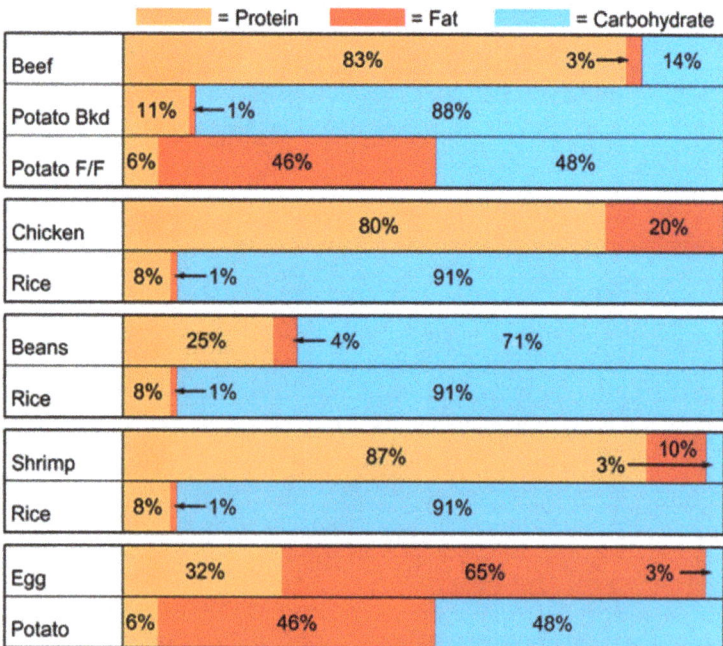

	= Protein	= Fat	= Carbohydrate
Beef	83%	3%→	14%
Potato Bkd	11% ←1%	88%	
Potato F/F	6% 46%	48%	
Chicken	80%	20%	
Rice	8% ←1%	91%	
Beans	25% ←4%	71%	
Rice	8% ←1%	91%	
Shrimp	87%	3%→	10%
Rice	8% ←1%	91%	
Egg	32%	65%	3% →
Potato	6% 46%	48%	

(These percentages are grams per unit of volume.)

Salad type vegetables are less complex in that they need less specific pH control and can compatibly withstand the pH changes in the stomach required by more complex foods. Once the food has reached the small intestine, the pH needs to be rather constant at around 7.4 because the next stop is the blood, which must be maintained at 7.4 pH.

- Planning meals so that foods mix in the small intestine (rice for lunch and beans for supper) and not in the stomach at the same time may provide the body with the necessary amino acids to be able to construct a "complete" protein. Remember that the reconstruction process does not begin until the amino acids get into the cell (from the blood) and then if and only if the proper anabolic (reconstruction) enzymes (vitamins) are available.
- Please refer to this **HUMAN MACHINE BOOK** series and my web site www.thehumanmachine.com for supplement suggestions.

Reference material:
FOOD COMBINING MAKE EASY by Herbert M. Shelton, N.D.
FIT FOR LIFE by Harvey and Marilyn Diamond
EAT RIGHT FOR YOUR BLOOD TYPE by Peter D'Adamo
THE METABOLIC TYPING DIET by William Wolcott

- When we misuse and abuse our bodies by putting things into it that are not compatible with the system as described above, there are consequences.

Pain is the body's method of getting our attention. If we do not make the necessary adjustments in our behavior, the message (pain) gets louder until we do finally act. But by then we have typically fallen into recognizable **ache and pain profiles**, which Western medicine puts labels on and usually tries to anesthetize the symptoms with drugs and surgery, which in turn causes more pain and discomfort over the long haul. (See the chapter on **"Ache and Pain Profiles"** in Volume II of **THE HUMAN MACHINE BOOK**.)

Some of us insist on peak efficiency from our body, while others are not that concerned with "the best". Those of us that want to ensure that this machine (our body) functions well without aches and pains, will necessarily have to expend more time and energy on providing "premium fuel". Those of us that choose not to pay that much attention to the quality of fuel and maintenance procedures, will consequently end up experiencing premature degeneration, resulting in some form of discomfort, aches, and pains. Then there are some of us that will avoid all the misery by dying early.

I strongly suggest that you take the time to visit a few "old folks homes" before you decide on which course of action to take with your own life. You can then see the results of toxic food choices.

OLD IS WHEN...
"Getting a little action" means you
don't need to take any fiber today.

Toxins Create Dis - Ease

The body will attempt to remove the poisons created by defective digestion. This toxin removal procedure is what we experience as symptoms of **"dis - ease"**. Flus and colds and allergies and skin eruptions are the body's attempt to remove a toxin.

A **toxin** is described as **ANYTHING** that will interfere with or curtail any or all of the following activities:

- Ingestion
- Digestion
- Assimilation
- Circulation
- Absorption
- Excretion
- Sensitivity to environment
- Reproduction

Sometimes this toxin removal process employs the assistance of germs and viruses to help break down and "eat up" toxic residue in the tissues. It's important to realize that germs **do not cause** disease, they are the **result** of dis – ease. Dr. Ryke Hammer, a German physician, explains this phenomenon quite thoroughly in his "unique" approach to medicine called German New Medicine. (www.germannewmedicine.ca>.

Germs – Nature's Little Undertakers

Nature's little undertakers are always present everywhere inside and outside our bodies. They exist to clean up our messes. That's what they do for a living. They just "hang around" waiting for us to "throw them a bone". But in reality, we "throw" them much more that "a bone".

Because of our total lack of education and knowledge of how our bodies work, and the types of foods that we do and do not put into our bodies, most of us have created a paradise for these little critters. The job that they were designed by Nature to do is to clean up the "crumbs" that others leave behind. But in this case we leave the crumbs IN our behind as well as every other spare space in our bodies.

When our behavior results in undigested and rotting food residue collecting in our connective tissue and organs, the "microscopic mop brigade" comes to the rescue. When we supply them with abundant food (toxic residue), they start raising families. Don't forget that every life form excretes its waste.

Because these little critters live inside our bodies, they have no choice but to excrete their waste into our sewer system. When their numbers are low, our system can handle the extra trash. But when they have plenty to eat (rotting material), their numbers grow rapidly, quickly overloading our trash removal system.

We are supposed to live in balance and harmony with them, but when their numbers start to overwhelm our immune system, our bodies go into "invasion alert" status. This includes calling out the "National Guard" (white blood cells) and opening up all dumping ports (mucus production, diarrhea, nausea, sweat) and turning up the thermostat (fever) to control and evict the little darlings.

Once balance (homeostasis) has been reestablished, everyone goes back to a harmonious life as usual. Your **"disease"** has been "cured".

This is a critical concept:

When two warring parties are equal in every way, there is a "stand-off". Nothing happens. There is a stalemate.

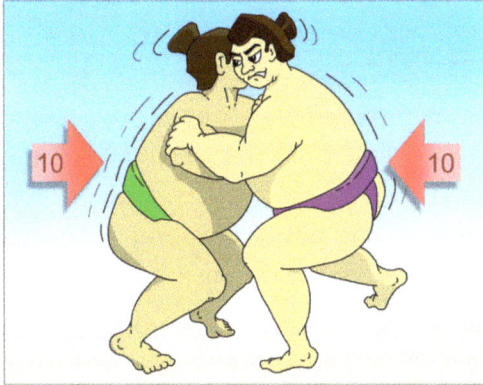

When one side is stronger than the other, the weaker one gets killed. We have to balance the parties in this "war" for territory (our bodies).

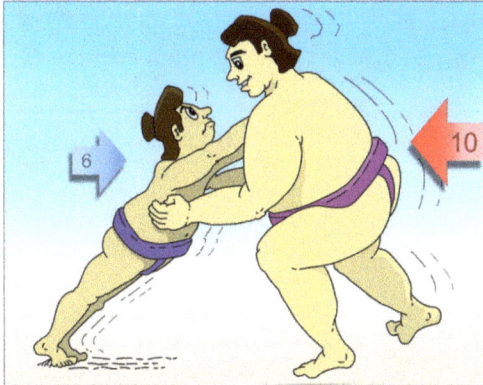

When there is a danger of the microbes getting the upper hand, and our immune system is not strong enough to resist, then we need to go to "war" and "kill the enemy" ... or at least reduce its numbers.

When our immune system is in great shape, we need not fear the microbe population. They will stay in their place until we offer them unlimited food supply. They are opportunists. They will then "go forth and multiply".

Digestion System Function

In a healthy body, starches begin the digestion process in the mouth. The food then passes through the esophagus to the stomach. The gastro-esophageal valve, which is located right where the stomach meets the esophagus, opens and lets the food into the upper part of the stomach.

Failure or leakage of this valve causes food mixed with stomach acids to leak back up into the esophagus causing a burning sensation in the middle of the chest. Western medicine refers to this condition as GERD (Gastro-Esophageal-Reflux-Disease). We'll come back to this subject further along in this text.

The starches (which are alkaline) will continue digesting in the upper part of the stomach for a short period of time, usually from 30 minutes to an hour or so, depending on what type and how much food was consumed. The protein (which is acid) in the meal that was just eaten will now trigger a reaction in the stomach that starts the production of Hydrochloric acid.

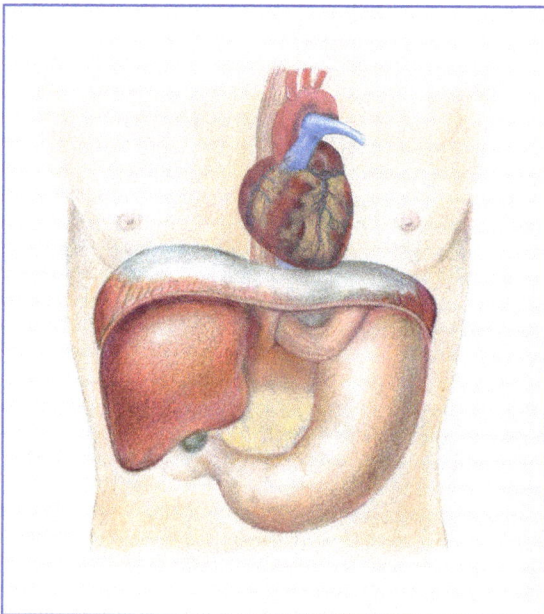

Hydrochloric Acid (HCl)

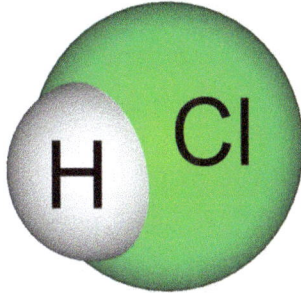

Hydrochloric acid (HCl) is a molecule made up of an atom of Hydrogen and an atom of Chlorine. The Hydrogen "shares" its electron with the Chlorine that is naturally missing one electron in its outer electron shell. (See Step 1)

However the Chlorine atom is bigger in size than the Hydrogen atom and, like any bully, hangs on to the shared electron more tightly than the Hydrogen does. (See Step 2)

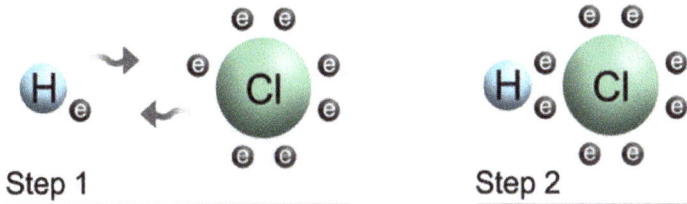

Step 1

Step 2

The above process can also be written like this :

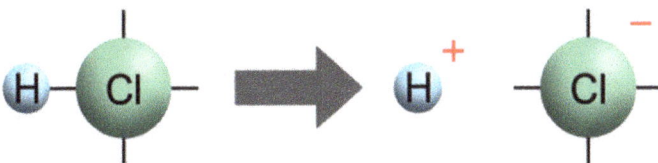

The hydrogen atom then can "lose" its electron to the Chlorine bully and the Hydrogen atom becomes a Hydrogen "ion" (an electrically unbalanced atom). The Hydrogen ion now carries a positive charge and the solution is now considered an acid.

For simplicity sake, if you had a bucket of Hydrogen atoms all missing their electron (positive electrical charge), you would have a bucket of very strong acid. If you had a bucket of Hydrogen atoms each with extra electrons (negative electrical charge), you would have a bucket of a strong alkaline solution. (For you chemists out there, I'm keeping this concept real simple.)

Without getting seriously mired down in the actual chemistry of digestion, let me just say that without HCl, adequate digestion and overall health is virtually impossible.

There are seven major activities that happen in the stomach with adequate supplies of HCl. If any one (or more) of these functions is disturbed and/or curtailed, serious health issues will develop over time.

First: HCl is necessary to stimulate the closing of the gastro-esophageal (LES) valve. If this valve does not close properly, food will back up into the throat. This is contrary to the popular belief that too much acid exists in the stomach and therefore the remedy for "heartburn" is to neutralize the stomach acid with an "anti-acid" pill or preparation.

Actually by consuming one or two tablespoons of apple cider vinegar before meals, the problem will usually resolve. There are worst-case scenarios that will be discussed further along in this text, but try this first.

Second: HCl is necessary to suspend the rotting process in the stomach until the digestive enzymes can start to break the food down. If you've ever bruised an apple, I'm sure that you have observed that it will turn brown and start to decompose within minutes. This is because every living thing has enzymes in it that are used to break the thing back down into earth elements from whence it came. When the living thing is damaged, its own "destruction enzymes" are released and the substance literally digests itself … it starts to rot.

The chewing process is designed to "bruise" and crush a piece of food so that the "break-down" enzymes are released to help in the digestion process.

I must emphasize here that this phenomenon takes place with RAW food, not cooked food. Heat distorts the shape of the enzyme and it no longer can "unlock" the bonds between the food molecules.

If you eat cooked food, there are no natural enzymes left in the food to assist the digestion process and the pancreas will need to work overtime creating the enzymes necessary to break the food down so that the body can assimilate the nutrients.

This extra "load" on the pancreas over time usually results in what western medicine calls diabetes. This is discussed in greater detail in Volume II.

After chewing and swallowing raw food such as an apple or a carrot, the natural enzymes from the apple will start to break it down very quickly. More than likely there will be other food in the stomach along with the apple that will require a longer time to be broken down enough to pass to the small intestine.

The HCl will suspend the rotting process until all the food is ready to proceed. Meat and other forms of flesh many times are not chewed as thoroughly as other food and will sit in the stomach in clumps. The outer edges will start to digest, but the inner parts will start to decompose. The HCl will suspend the rotting process while helping to break down the connective tissue of the muscle meat that you just ate, thereby assisting the enzyme, pepsin, to digest the protein.

Third: HCl is necessary to convert the relatively inert pepsinogen into pepsin. Pepsin is a protein-digesting enzyme. Pepsin starts the digestion of protein in the stomach. The walls of the stomach secrete a pepsin precursor called pepsinogen … pepsin – o – gen. The pepsinogen will not start to digest anything until HCl separates the "pepsin" from the "gen". In addition, HCl is necessary for Vitamin B-12 absorption. Lack of B-12 results in what Western Medicine calls pernicious anemia (lack of oxygen). Without adequate oxygen, the metabolic process is impaired giving rise to feelings of exhaustion and low energy.

Therefore destroying HCl in the stomach with anti-acids will guarantee that protein will rot in the stomach instead of being digested. We will discuss the repercussions later in this text.

Fourth: HCl is necessary to kill bacteria that come into the digestive tract on the food that we eat. Helicobacter Pylori bacteria infection is thought (by western medicine) to cause stomach ulcers.

In actual fact, H-Pylori cannot exist in the stomach with adequate concentrations of HCl. Destroying the stomach acids with "antacids" invites not only H-Pylori, but a whole host of disturbances that will be enumerated throughout this text.

Fifth: HCl is necessary to "chelate" minerals so that they can gain access to the blood through the small intestine. There are uptake structures in the small intestine for proteins (amino acids), simple sugars, and fatty acids.

There is no such structure in the small intestine to take in minerals. The mineral must play "Trojan Horse" to get into the blood. A protein must wrap itself around the mineral to take it into the blood.

A mineral is a smooth sided crystal. There are no "handles" for the protein to hang on to the mineral. HCl etches "handles" into the sides of the mineral crystal so that the protein can carry the mineral into the blood through the protein-access openings in the small intestine. (See the electron stealing process discussion above.)

Without HCl in the stomach, minerals cannot get into the blood to provide the center structures for building enzymes and hormones. Minerals are also critical for the function of muscles and nerves, especially the brain.

If HCl is inhibited and/or curtailed, vital functions of the body are in jeopardy. As soon as stored minerals are used up, the body will start to cannibalize itself and a state of disintegration and/or **degenerative dis – ease** develops.

There is *some* mineral absorption in the large intestine, but the stomach needs to be functioning adequately to create the proper environment in the large intestine to allow mineral absorption to take place.

Sixth: HCl is necessary to trigger the opening of the pyloric valve (from the stomach to the small intestine). The stomach muscles churn the contents and mix the HCl thoroughly with the food.

The pyloric valve will open and let the food (now called chyme) into the small intestine when the valve senses that the concentration of HCl has reached a predetermined threshold.

For example, when just fruit is in the stomach, the acid bias on the pyloric valve is low and the valve will open with minimum squeezing pressure from the churning of the stomach muscles.

But when protein is in the stomach, the HCl requirement is elevated to be able to process the protein properly. This raises the bias on the pyloric valve to stay closed until the protein food in the stomach is adequately mixed with HCl to ensure thorough break down of the protein.

Once again, if the HCl is neutralized (by pharmaceutical anti- acids or alkaline from starchy food), the valve becomes "confused" and will open at the wrong time and allow undigested food into the small intestine, which will result in more chemical stress that results in allergies and other functional disturbances.

In a properly functioning stomach, the food will be mixed with HCl in order to open the pyloric valve. The food then moves into the duodenum or the first third of the small intestine where there is no protection from the acid from the stomach.

Seventh: An adequate concentration of HCl in the stomach is necessary to signal the pancreas to produce Sodium Bicarbonate (NaHCO3), which is a buffer or base, which is supposed to neutralize the acid coming from the stomach.

The stomach is insulated from HCl by a layer of mucus that lines the entire stomach. The small intestine does not have this protection and will be chemically burned if the acid from the stomach is allowed to pass into it.

Therefore, if HCl concentration in the stomach is inadequate, low (or no) levels of NaHCO3 (Sodium bicarbonate) will be produced from the pancreas. This will result in some acid from the stomach passing into the small intestine unbuffered.

The stomach acid will literally chemically burn the small intestine, destroying the villi (the nutrient uptake mechanisms in the small intestine), creating holes and scar tissue, resulting in what western medicine calls "leaky gut".

This situation creates a number of down-stream problems. The villi in the small intestine are designed to absorb nutrients from digestion into the blood. With the number of functional villi in the small intestine reduced from the acid burn, fewer nutrients can enter the blood. In addition, the damaged small intestine tissue will now allow complex proteins into the blood stream. The villi in the small intestine are designed to allow only single amino acids into the blood.

More complex amino acid groups can sneak into the blood through larger openings in the damaged villi. Any complex proteins entering the blood from the small intestine that do not carry a "self- identity tag" (DNA) will now trigger an "allergic" response.

Allergy symptoms are the body's attempt to get rid of potentially dangerous "foreign" protein molecules. The body will attempt to dump the "foreign protein" either through the mucus membranes or through the skin. Skin rashes and mucus discharges are the body's garbage overflow.

Look at babies. Does this phenomenon start to make any sense with respect to constant runny gooey noses and wax plugged ears and blocked eustation tubes? Does it cause you to reflect on what you are putting into their little mouths? Please refer to the REVERSE ENGINEERING chapter in Volume II for what kinds of food to feed babies and when to introduce them.

But there is another more ominous result of the leaky gut syndrome.

Candida Albicans

The small intestine typically harbors a yeast/fungus called candida albicans. This is a natural resident in the small intestine that helps in the digestion of starches. The body's immune system, along with strict intestinal pH control, keeps the growth of this fungus within acceptable limits, so that it stays in the small intestine.

But when the natural balance of the body is disturbed, the body's immune system cannot keep the candida where it belongs. The "weeds" (candida) will grow out of control and take over the entire alimentary tract.

The candida growth can be seen in the stool and in the throat and on the tongue as a white and sometimes yellowish coating that has a very distinct breath odor. Western medicine refers to this condition as "thrush" and prescribes anti-biotic and anti-fungal agents. But the worst is yet to come.

The "leaky gut" now allows the candida that should be restricted to the small intestine to enter the blood stream. This is much more problematic than overgrowth of candida in the digestive tract.

This "systemic candida" now infects the entire body. Everywhere the blood goes, the candida now has access. This means that all of the organs, including the liver and the kidneys and the brain, have been invaded by the candida fungus.

Keep in mind that nothing happens without a reason.

If complex proteins are allowed to enter the blood, they will clog up the lymphatic system and negatively affect the absorption of nutrients into the cells.

These complex proteins cannot enter the cells because of their size and structure. They therefore continue to circulate through the blood and lymphatic system and eventually deposit themselves in the tissues resulting in aches and pains.

Western medicine then puts labels on the pain like fibromyalgia, or bursitis, or arthritis, or carpal tunnel syndrome. Remember that we have discussed the fact that protein as well as any organic material has a useful "life" after which they will decompose in a warm, dark, moist place.

As this "foreign" protein looks for a place to hide, the body allows "Nature's little undertakers", bacteria and fungi, to pass through the same openings in the small intestine that the complex proteins slipped through into the blood supply.

As in all natural processes, that which does not get digested properly, will be broken down by germs and fungi … putrefaction and fermentation. That's exactly what Nature intended for these little critters.

"**Nature is <u>always</u> in balance**".

This process of systemic candida proliferation is one of the prerequisite conditions for cancer tumors to develop. Tulio Simoncini, M.D. has observed that lung "cancer tumors" can be dissolved by administering sodium bicarbonate solution to the affected tissues.

His observations may be correct, but, in my opinion, his conclusions are flawed. His photos of the "cancer colony" disappearing with the application of sodium bicarbonate solution are showing the destruction of the candida nests that have been drawn to the area to "eat up" the cell proliferation ("cancer"). See www.germannewmedicine.ca for an in depth discussion on how the body uses germs (especially the tuberculosis bacteria) and fungi to "eat up" the tumor growth and bring the body back to homeostasis.

Linda Allen has written a very informative book on candida called "Yeast Infection No More". I highly recommend this book if you have a chronic candida overgrowth problem.

For improving the overall efficiency and optimal health at the cellular level, that is, improving the mechanical function of each cell in your body, check out <thehumanamchine.teamasea.com>. In order to assist the body to purge the invading candida, and other contaminates, by the way, from the blood and tissues, I have found that a proteolytic enzyme taken in between meals will speed up the process. There are a number of brands of proteolytic (protein digesting) enzymes on the market that will do the job. You can take two or three capsules of these proteolytic enzymes at least three times per day, preferably a half hour or so before meals (empty stomach). Taking the enzymes on an empty stomach, will not waist the enzymes digesting your food. They will get into the blood stream to digest the protein particles in your tissues that are causing your fibromyalgia pains and systemic candida.

Germs and Fungi

Have you ever noticed that if a cop pulls you over on the highway for a tail light out or maybe you were weaving a little on the road, that your whole car and its occupants and contents are open for scrutiny? They're going to find all sorts of interesting things in your car that you would rather they not find.

Germs and fungi do exactly the same thing. When the call goes out that there is a problem somewhere in the system, the little undertakers are released to find the problem and obliterate it.

The problem is that they will keep on looking, just like the nosey cop with your car. And you can rest assured that they (the fungi and germs) will find something else that needs cleaning out. And we now have a "systemic infection".

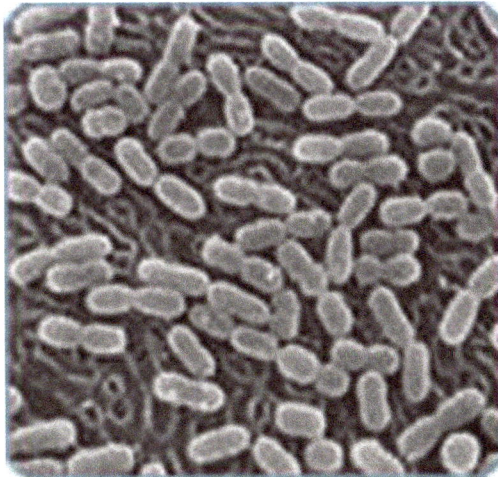

If the body's immune system is not strong enough to keep these guys in check while they're cleaning up your mess, and if you are harboring more doo-doo in your system in other places, these little critters will seek out the extra doo-doo (their food supply) and continue to proliferate.

Tumors / Cancer

In addition to the undigested protein in the blood, if the body has developed a tumor or other growth or degeneration process, the little critter detail will be dispatched to help to restore balance by attempting to "eat up" the tumor also. These tumor sites and defective, contaminated tissue areas become excellent breeding grounds for the Candida, bacteria, and viruses.

This is what Hulda Clark, N.D., PhD. and Tulio Simoncini, M.D. discovered. This is also what Royal Raymond Rife saw in his famous microscope back in the 1930's. He quickly gained the reputation of being able to "cure" cancer with his "Rife Frequency Generator".

Gaston Naesson created a similar microscope and developed his "7-14-X" intra-lymphaticly injectable solution that he has also used very successfully in Montreal Canada for "tumor" growth.

These "candida nests" if given the proper local and global emotional, energetic, and basic survival chemistry environment as discovered by Ryke Hamer, M.D., (www.germannewmedicine.ca) can trigger an uncontrolled cell growth pattern that we call "**cancer**".

A cancer cell is by definition a normal body cell that has mutated from its original aerobic function to an anaerobic function. The detailed mechanics of DNA warping is immaterial at this point.

The bottom line here is that the normal body cell will function and stay alive by using oxygen. It's important to emphasize here that an oxygen molecule has a negative charge bias, which is alkaline in nature. (See page 61).

If something happens to cut off or limit the supply of oxygen to the cell, the cell will employ a built-in survival technique and switch to anaerobic (without oxygen) behavior to stay alive. This is a normal natural self-defense procedure that the cell employs to stay alive and viable. This anaerobic mode utilizes sugar for metabolism instead of oxygen. Sugar is acidic.

The sugar distorts the DNA chain and the mutation has begun. We now have a **cancer cell** population beginning. (See "CANCER" in VOL II.)

If we could find the *original irritant* that caused the first cell to switch from aerobic to anaerobic behavior, we would be able to stop the progress of the tumor ... and, by the way, return the defective cell to its normal natural aerobic function.

We will be discussing three modes of irritation that would cause a cell to mutate into a cancer cell. I might add, at this point, that there are cancer cells all over the healthy body all the time. The strong immune system in a healthy body will keep these rogue cells under control. A suppressed immune system cannot police the area adequately to maintain equilibrium and homeostasis, and degenerative dis - eases will ensue.

I would like to emphasize at this point that along with having a good rich soil base and an adequate water supply and a compatible supportive climate, a "seed" is still necessary for a plant to grow. Even though all the supportive environmental conditions are present in the body to create a cancer tumor growth, there still needs to be a "seed" event to stimulate the cells to an abnormal growth pattern.

This "seed" event is explained effectively and competently by Riker Hammer, M.D. in his concept of GERMAN NEW MEDICINE. Dr. Hammer explains that the brains of all animals are programmed for survival. (See my discussion of INSTICTIVE / VOLITIONAL behavior in Volume I of this series.) According to Dr. Hammer, if the animal (including humans) experiences an unexpected emotional shock event, the brain will register the event in a specific geographic location in the brain.

This specific group of brain cells will reflex to a particular part of the body of the animal that can "respond" to the potential threat to the survival of the animal. This event will result in either the abnormal growth of, or deterioration of, a specific part of the body that will encourage survival.

According to Dr. Hammer, this reactionary survival behavior is temporary and the body will return to "normal" life activity with the resolution of the presenting conflict. This resolution behavior is a natural preprogrammed process.

An example of this phenomenon is breast cancer. If a woman experiences a perceived "emotional shock" concerning her "nest" or children, the left breast will be affected. With respect to the basic hard-wire animal survival instinct, the breast of the female is designed to nurture and feed the baby. If the baby's health is perceived to be threatened, the automatic feedback loop to the brain is triggered to pump out more milk to feed the sick baby. This is accomplished by creating more cells in the breast as soon as possible to create more milk to heal the sick baby ... cancer tumor.

Keep in mind that this is a subconscious automatic hard-wire feedback loop designed for survival of the organism. There are many more complex issues concerning this process, but this is as simple as I can state it in this limited space. This is an exciting breakthrough in the understanding of ease and dis – ease.

The information that I am presenting in this book series is consistent with and supportive of Dr. Hammer's discoveries. My addition to the scenario that Dr. Hammer presents is that our present "modern" artificial life style creates a pre-loading stress condition that exaggerates the effects of the "survival response" and sabotages the natural healing process.

In this modern "civilized" world, sickness is BIG business. And because cancer is BIG business, the "cure" for cancer will always be "just around the corner". "We're almost there".

"They" have to keep the game going. If they find a "cure", the game is over and the mega-business will collapse. There are unbelievable profits being made by the drug companies and the "medical machine" in the pursuit of "the cure" for cancer, diabetes, heart disease, and whatever other "disease" that they can come up with that they decide needs a war against it.

In the mean time, many people will die an unnecessarily expensive, painful, and agonizing death. We will ALL die eventually. We do not have conscious control over the time of our stay here on this planet, but we DO have ultimate control over the quality of that time.

I'd be willing to bet a considerable sum of money though that even after understanding the root cause of cancer and other tumors in the body, a great number of folks will continue on with the same behavior as before. This means that many people will probably still create a cancer and/or cause an existing one to continue to grow until it consumes them because "change" is scary and/or difficult.

Once again …

"You've got what you've got because you did what you did.

If you continue to do what you did, you'll continue to get what you've got."

I say this because most people will not accept the responsibility for their own actions and behaviors. AND cancer, along with all these other degenerative dis - eases that seem to "attack" us when we're not looking, are ALL the result of behavior.

Behaviors have consequences.

Being a "victim" is what we are all taught to do. As I explain in Volume I, "I hope this presentation motivates you to action". I'm not going to hold my breath though, but I DO have hope. It is the purpose of this book to show that *we have choices for behavior.*

Out of the numbers of those folks who are reading this book, a few of you have realized that we have already discussed the cause of cancer. For those who haven't made the connection yet, let's lay it out in specific detail. I'm going to repeat myself here, but I want to create a schematic diagram or road map so that we can follow the steps mechanically from

Stress to Indigestion to Cancer

The three scenarios that I mentioned that <u>may</u> result in anaerobic cell behavior leading to cancer are:

1) Traumatic repetitive injuries
2) Microscopic invaders including viruses, bacteria, fungus
3) Chemicals

Any or all of these situations may be present and no cancer will develop unless there is an emotional or psychological (belief system) survival-threat triggering-event. See above paragraphs describing the concept of GERMAN NEW MEDICINE.

Can you see the "elephant in the room" yet? All these researchers are discovering valid factual data. But the problem goes much deeper than one or two observable factoids.

The situation is similar to the belief that the rooster crowing in the morning brings the sun up. Certainly every time that the rooster wakes up and crows, the sun rises. "It must be a causal relationship". The rooster must certainly bring up the sun because absolutely every time the rooster crows in the morning, daylight follows. But what happens if we kill the rooster or put him in a box where no one can hear him? Will the sun come up?

Truly the bacteria and fungi that are observed in and around troubled flesh **ARE NOT** the problem. They are trying to help you *solve* the problem.

The difficulty arises when you cannot control the population of your helpers and they literally eat you out of house and home. Sometimes when the clean-up squad gains the upper hand, we can employ a little help in the control department with limited, and hopefully natural, herbal antibiotics to bring the situation under control. I emphasize the word "little" here.

If you completely obliterate the helpers, there is a temporary cease-fire, but the "bad guys" are the first ones back on the scene to continue to stress your immune system and exacerbate the problem.

PHIL SELINSKY, N.D.

The "good guys" are bacteria that utilize oxygen in their metabolic activity. They are referred to as "aerobic". The "bad guys" are bacteria that have learned to survive without oxygen. These are "anaerobic" bacteria.

Virtually all detrimental bacteria are anaerobic, including cells in the body that have also "learned" to survive without oxygen. These are **cancer tumor** cells. Oxygen is their nemesis. A "pharmaceutical (chemical) antibiotic" (against life) kills all bacteria ... good and bad.

Sometimes in certain circumstances, big pharmaceutical and surgical guns are necessary to resolve a crisis situation. I would not be here today to write this book if it were not for Western medicine's "big guns" when I was 13. But anything to extremes is dangerous.

The "good guys" help kill the "bad guys" and keep you in homeostasis – balance – health. A "natural antibiotic" utilizes oxygen to kill only "anaerobic" bacteria, which includes mutated body cells ... **cancer tumors**.

- Nicotine
- Caffeine
- Alcohol
- Refined Sugar
- Refined Flour
- Dairy Products (anything produced from or with milk)
- Drugs (pharmaceutical as well as street/recreational drugs)

These are ALL acid-forming substances. Cut them OUT of your life NOW. Cancer cells thrive in an acid environment. Oxygen is alkalizing. See my web site (www.thehumanmachine.com) for more suggestions and ideas on sources of oxygen if you are experiencing a problem with tumor growth or arthritic pains.

The Butterfly in the Cocoon

In addition, remember the story of the butterfly in the cocoon? An individual, walks by a butterfly in a cocoon struggling to break out into the world.

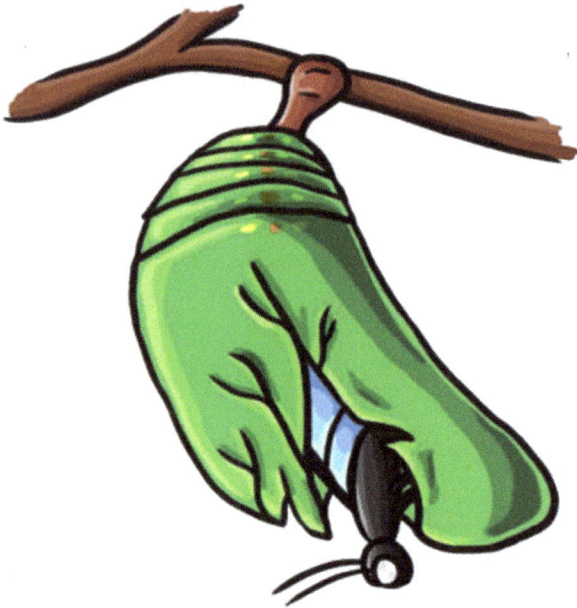

After watching the struggle for a while, the individual decides to "help" the butterfly in its struggle to be born and cuts the cocoon. But instead of taking flight, the crumpled butterfly tumbles to the ground unable to either get up or to fly. Why? …

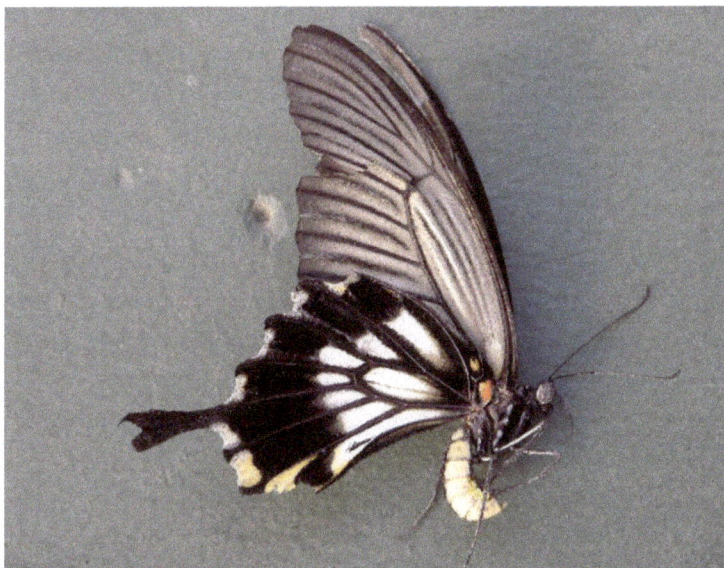

Because the butterfly did not have to struggle to get out of the cocoon, it did not get a chance to get strong enough to withstand the challenges of life and it dies. Our immune system has the same challenge.

In our "modern" society we try to "help" our immune system to overcome the "infection" by taking antibiotics. This does not allow the immune system the opportunity to get strong enough to truly and emphatically repel the army of microbes that are actually there to help the body get rid of the trash that YOU put there in the first place with your injudicious eating habits.

Most importantly, cleaning up the area, which includes physical internal hygiene (digestion) and emotional and spiritual balancing (stress) many times requires changing life style and behavior.

Just like hiring your house cleaning out to someone else who doesn't know what's important to you, the "little critter clean-up brigade" may inadvertently end up damaging some useful parts and pieces of your living space … your body. The key here is **<u>do</u> <u>not</u>** continue to attempt to live in a cesspool and expect the critter population to forget where you live.

Pancreas Disturbances

We've discussed some of the ramifications of improper digestion due to a problem with a lack of, or low HCl production. There are more low HCl problems that we'll address later in this text, but first we should also discuss the pancreas issue.

Previously, we mentioned that NaHCO3 production in the pancreas is affected by HCl concentration in the stomach. The glandular secretions from the pancreas include NaHCO3, insulin, and digestive enzymes.

When one part of the pancreas is disturbed, everything else is also affected. This means that when we have suppressed or depressed NaHCO3 output, for whatever reason, insulin and digestive enzymes are also restricted.

Low insulin production, allows high blood sugar, which is by definition, diabetes, and low digestive enzyme production, which results in gas and bloating and cramping.

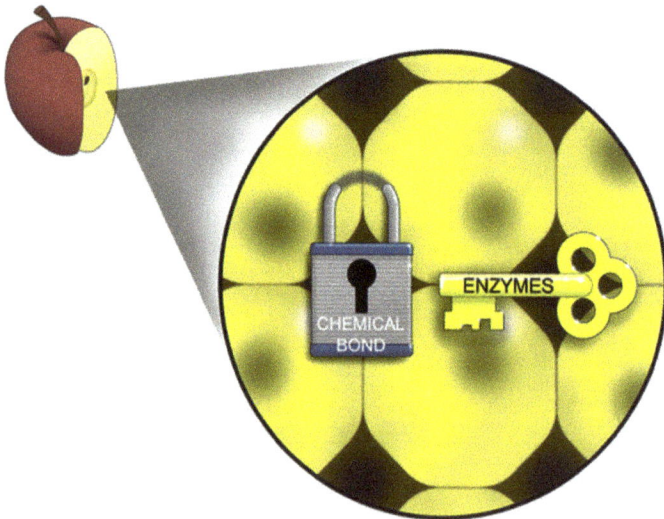

PHIL SELINSKY, N.D.

Enzymes are chemical keys that unlock the chemical bonds that hold the molecules of food material together in their shape and form.

In addition, we eat cooked food that has had all its natural enzymes destroyed from the heat.

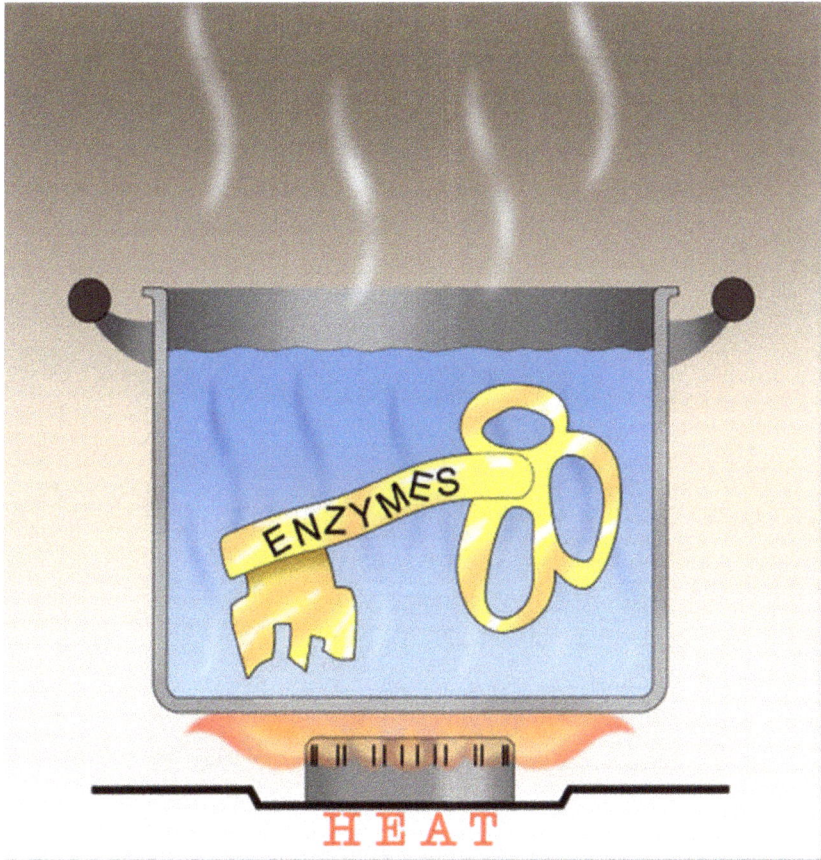

Remember that heat distorts the configuration of protein. Enzymes are proteins. Enzymes need their special shape to act as a chemical key to unlock the bonds that hold food material together. When you heat the enzyme, you change its shape and therefore render it useless to break your food down.

The food material now will putrefy in a warm dark moist place causing gas and bloating and intestinal spasms, which we feel as abdominal cramps. Further down the road in the large intestine, the problem continues.

Large Intestine

The major job of the large intestine is to dehydrate the material coming from the small intestine. The body is a conservative and efficient machine. It takes advantage of any and all structures or mechanisms for multiple purposes.

The water that has been used in the digestion process is now taken back up into the blood stream from the large intestine. This process is accomplished by wrapping lymph ducts around the large intestine much like tree roots wrap around a sewer pipe.

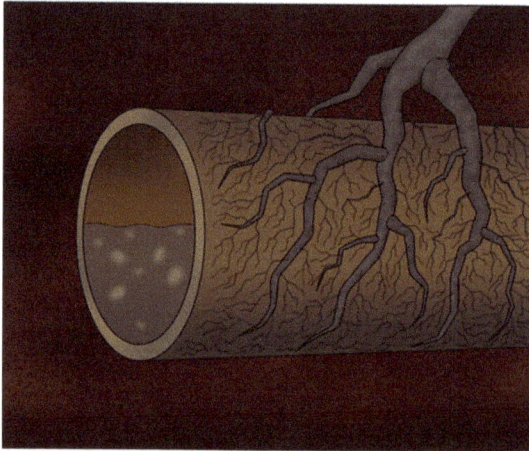

Through the process of osmosis, the lymphatic tissue absorbs the water from the large intestine. Then the lymph system eventually dumps into the blood system.

Please keep in mind that when you pour water through coffee grounds, what ends up in your cup is not pure water. We observe the same phenomenon in the large intestine.

When we have cesspool water in the large intestine, can you guess what gets sucked up into the lymphatic system? If we load up the lymphatic system with rotting doo-doo from the large intestine, a number of nasty things will begin to happen.

Lymphatic Contamination

One big problem develops from the fact that the lower pelvis area is densely populated with lymphatic plumbing. And the reproductive organs also "live" in the same drainage neighborhood and get bathed in this cesspool of contaminated lymphatic fluid.

The tissues of the uterus and ovaries and bladder in females and the prostate and bladder in males get chemically irritated from the contaminated lymph fluid, and over time can become chronically infected. (See GERMS AND FUNGI on page 83.) This chronic irritation, can and often does result in uncontrolled tissue growth (tumors).

Chronic Interstitial Cystitis is a condition that usually develops in females along with Chronic Vaginitis and frequent Vaginal Fungus (Candida). Remember our discussion on "anaerobic" life forms?

The chemical contamination of the tissues of the colon occurs over time (years) from improper food combinations and preservatives and food additives. These chemicals anesthetize and retard the peristalsis (contractions) and absorption of fluids from the colon so that the material spends more time than necessary in the colon and consequently putrefies and contaminates the lymphatic system, which leads to the above described conditions.

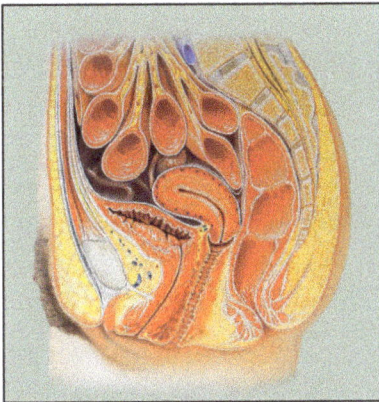

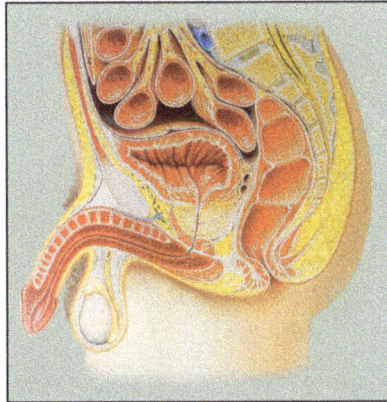

Spleen – Immune System

In addition, the contaminated lymph now flows to the spleen. The spleen is the largest lymph organ in the body. The spleen is also the recycling plant for old broken down red blood cells. If the spleen becomes irritated and encumbered, the blood will be affected.

The recycling of red blood cells releases bilirubin into the blood. The liver then uses the bilirubin to make bile. Proper bile constitution is necessary to both stimulate the large intestine peristalsis and to emulsify fats that are further digested so that they can be used to create hormones.

The energy that drives the spleen also is responsible for the distribution of fluids throughout the body. (Please refer to Volume II for a more in depth explanation of the energy that drives all the organs.)

Dry eyes, dry mouth, dry vagina, and low seminal fluid volume are all functions of the affected spleen, which in turn affects the energy circuit that drives all the other functions that are mentioned here.

The opposite is also true. Runny eyes, excess saliva, excessive vaginal secretions (outside of sexual arousal), wet hands, wet feet are all excesses of the spleen/pancreas energy circuit.

The symptoms of excess listed here are usually the responsibility of the pancreas function. This situation can typically be traced to too much sugar or the inability to digest or process sugar or sugary foods, which is an enzyme deficit.

Once again, we find ourselves back to the stomach as the original "bad guy". If the stomach is malfunctioning, all other systems will be affected.

The liver is the chemical factory in the body. It has hundreds of chemical responsibilities in the body in addition to "cleaning" the toxins out of the blood and monitoring fat and sugar metabolism.

When the liver is overloaded with blood contamination coming from the large intestine, this takes priority over all other functions. If your body is overcome with toxins and poisons, you could die. So everything including sugar and fat metabolism is put "on hold" until the body can effectively neutralize the poisons.

(Reread the definitions of "toxins" or "poisons" on page #71 of this text. See also the ACHE AND PAIN profiles in Volume II for the body aches and pains associated with certain organ and organ systems.)

Please keep in mind that all of this "malfunction syndrome" is the result of the problem with the stomach. If the stomach is injured or damaged or the energy supply is inadequate, food will not digest properly and will putrefy at the beginning of the alimentary canal.

This means that by the time the food reaches the large intestine, most of it has putrefied already and has gathered a whole convention of anaerobic bacteria that feeds on rotting material.

This stresses the immune system. Most importantly, since most of the food has putrefied, there is little "real live food" that can be used for fuel and construction and repair, further weakening the body's resistance to dis – ease.

IF YOU CANNOT DIGEST YOUR FOOD
YOU CANNOT REPAIR YOUR BODY!!!

Probiotics

Now you can start to see why **probiotics** are necessary for large intestine integrity. Probiotics (pro = for, bio = life) are microbes that are aerobic (oxygen users). They utilize oxygen for metabolism.

They eat the undigested protein in the large intestine and excrete an acid waste. This creates an acid bias in the large intestine to suspend the rotting process in the colon until the leftover material from digestion gets properly dehydrated.

This process may take maybe a day or so to complete. Remember that protein held in a warm, dark, moist place will rot.

Feces should not rot until it leaves the body. If it rots IN the body, the putrefying material gets into the lymphatic system and eventually into the blood.

The contamination from "anaerobic" (without oxygen) bacteria changes the pH bias in the large intestine, which encourages the growth of tumors.

In addition, if toxic material cannot exit through normal channels (normal regular defecation), it will find another way out. It may come out through the skin or through the lungs or through the mucus membranes.

Or it might "tunnel" through from the large intestine to the skin around the anal area in the form of a fissure, or a fistula, or a boil. (See Volume II for a discussion on the purpose of the appendix with respect to natural bacteria generation in the large intestine.)

Summary of the Mechanics of the Hiatal Hernia

As discussed earlier in this text, the original responsible agent or "bad guy" here is the genetically weak liver circuit that suppresses the connective tissue integrity, which allows a hernia of the tissue of the hiatus in the diaphragm to develop.

Once the hiatal hernia condition exists, frequently the stomach literally gets sucked up into and becomes pinched in the enlarged opening in the diaphragm. The damaged stomach becomes swollen and irritated and cannot produce the necessary enzymes and acids to properly begin the digestion of food. The tissue irritation spreads to the small intestine and then to the large intestine.

The ensuing inflammatory condition puts a stress on all sections of the alimentary tract including the vagus nerve, which enervates the entire digestive system as well as the heart and lungs.. As already discussed, the stomach, the small intestine, and the large intestine, each have their own power circuits along with their corresponding "reserve tank" muscle groups.

The energy that is robbed from the reserve tank muscles to run the overburdened digestive organs leads to all the muscle aches and pains and symptom profiles that we have discussed above.

If the stomach stays in the "pinched" condition, the symptoms cannot get better without intervention. In other words, nothing will change unless and until you get the stomach down out of the hole in the diaphragm, relieving the physical irritation.

You can live inside of a health food store and eat the "best" food on the planet and have beautiful positive thoughts, and dress in pink robes, and meditate 23 hours a day, but you will still experience a life full of discomfort and pain if the stomach remains physically damaged from the hernia.

To solve this problem,

YOU <u>MUST</u> GET THE STOMACH OUT OF THE HOLE IN THE DIAPHRAGM.

There are a number of techniques and protocols that address this situation. In Part III, I list some of the effective practices that I have found that do, in fact, reduce the symptoms of Hiatal Hernia.

PART III

THE REMEDY

Structural vs Functional Hiatal Hernia

I have found that there are two types or phases of the Hiatal Hernia Syndrome phenomenon. The most serious type is the actual herniation of the diaphragm with the stomach physically up into the chest cavity as in the picture on page 24.

If you have a "**structural hiatal hernia**", physically pulling the stomach down is the only process that can actually work to relieve the nagging symptom profile.

If you have a "**functional hiatal hernia**" condition, it is possible to perform the practices and exercises that I have described below to actually relieve the symptoms without having to get your stomach "pulled".

It's quicker and more effective to just have it pulled, but if the stomach is not actually "trapped" in the diaphragm, the stretching exercises will work.

If you are suffering from a **structural hiatal hernia**, as opposed to a **functional hiatal hernia,** there is a visceral manipulation that can relieve this unfortunate situation. In plain English, the stomach MUST be physically pulled down out of the hole in the diaphragm and "taught" to stay down in order to relieve the chronic nagging symptoms and degenerative conditions that result from this condition.

There are a number of chiropractors and osteopaths like Theodore Baroody, D.C. (mentioned earlier), who have been performing different forms of manipulation over the years to pull the stomach down. Not all chiropractors or osteopaths have the knowledge and the experience to do this maneuver successfully. As a matter of fact, very few medical professionals in any discipline or specialty know how to treat a hiatal hernia outside of surgery. You'll have to search around for someone in your area that is at all familiar with the concept. I learned a procedure from an "old" osteopath back in 1977 that seems to do the job better than most of the chiropractic maneuvers that I've seen.

Early 1900's massage therapists and osteopathic physicians were trained in actual physical body contact and visceral manipulation techniques.

If you can find an osteopath in his or her 70's or older, they have been trained in how to move organs around to change body dynamics. The younger Nickie-New-Guys in the profession have been strongly influenced by the pharmaceutical industry and unfortunately will not be experienced enough in these techniques.

WARNING !!!!

There is a real danger of cracking a rib or snapping one rib over another when performing this **hiatal hernia** maneuver, so unless you are a professional practitioner, **DO NOT** try this at home without competent hands on instruction.

Attention Professionals !!!!

In order to pull the stomach down out of the hole in the diaphragm, you must get your fingers up under the rib cage in between the diaphragm and the stomach and pull down towards the feet. The two floating ribs are in danger of being snapped if you do not place your hands on the abdomen properly.

You must also create enough "slack" in the skin so that you do not cause the ribs to be pulled down by the abdominal muscle attachments on the ribs as your fingers push back along the surface of the diaphragm. This is what can cause rib damage. See picture on page 112.

It's tricky. But it CAN be done. It only takes a couple of seconds to perform, but it takes skill to know how and where to press and how much pressure to exert pulling the stomach out of the hole.

Another important issue is that of osteoporosis. If the person that you're working on has a fragile bone condition, **DO NOT DO THIS PROCEDURE UNLESS YOU HAVE BEEN TRAINED PROPERLY ... and even then, with severe osteoporosis, it's safer to use nutrition first and then attempt to move the stomach with the gentler "Polarity holding" procedure that I'll describe a few paragraphs down.**

Be especially alert for people who have been taking drugs like Fosamax, Boniva, Actonel, Micalcin, or similar pharmaceutical drug. The use of these drugs over time all result in old brittle bones that break easily rather than stimulating new flexible bone growth. (See the discussion on osteoporosis in Volume II.)

Some stomachs can be stubborn. Sometimes it can necessitate two or three tries, but eventually the stomach will come down to live where it should be. I have taught this technique to a few people so far. It's not something that just anyone can or should do.

This procedure may result in bruising of the abdominal muscles. If bruising results easily, load up on Vitamin K and C for a few days prior and take homeopathic Arnica (6, 12, or 30X will do) at least a week before and a week after.

Back to the general population ...

What You Can Do For Yourself

I must add at this point that the stomach may not necessarily have to actually be "in the hole" to elicit all these discomfort profiles that are associated with the **Hiatal Hernia Syndrome**.

The stomach can just be cramped and "contracted" up against the diaphragm due to stress, to cause you to experience the whole gamut of symptoms that you would feel if you had a full-blown x-ray verifiable hernia condition.

This gives rise to the frustration felt when you experience the tell-tale discomforts and symptoms of the classic **hiatal hernia profile**, but when you go to western medicine for an official diagnosis, they can't find anything. X-rays and endoscopies show nothing out of "normal".

You are labeled a "hypochondriac" and they prescribe antipsychotic drugs to "relax" you. Well, they are inadvertently on the right track by assuming that there may be an emotional or stress related component here, but they do not know how emotions or stress can cause your symptoms or what to do about it if they did know.

Certainly, the drugs will cause more problems down stream, which will lead to the "need" for more drugs, which will severely overload the liver, which will very often generate the feeling of wanting to blow your brains out because there seems to be no answer to your suffering (from western medicine, that is).

Spiritual, emotional, and/or physical stress can and often does result in digestive disturbance. Digestive disturbance, over time, WILL result in degenerative conditions that as we get older, will result in many aches and pains that most everyone seems to expect as part of aging.

I totally disagree with that particular projection and expected profile of aging. I've mentioned in Volumes I and II that this "machine" (our body) that we drive around in every day was designed to function **in** Nature **with** Nature, and that severe repercussions can be expected for violating Nature's laws.

The corollary of that is that if you follow Nature's laws, your body can be expected to "run" relatively trouble free (minus traumatic injuries, that is) for the duration of your stay here on this planet regardless of how many years that takes.

Pain is not necessary, but it is inevitable.

Stomach Muscle Spasms

The stomach is a muscular bag composed of a number of layers of muscles all contracting in different directions, allowing the stomach to be able to squeeze and churn food into a semi liquid paste called chyme, which then moves through the pyloric valve at the lower end of the stomach into the small intestine to continue the digestion process.

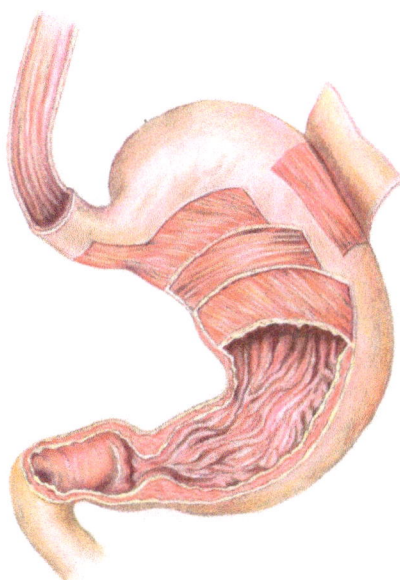

If these stomach muscles start to spasm or "Charlie horse" due to lack of minerals and/or dehydration, the spasming stomach muscles will put contraction stress on the esophagus and the diaphragm, resulting in some or all of the hiatal hernia symptoms. In addition, the spasming stomach muscles can squeeze and restrict more of the blood from the stomach muscle itself, resulting in more intense spasms and pain. See the Polarity holding technique a few paragraphs down on page 111.

At this point, the spasming stomach may squeeze some of the HCl from the stomach up through the lower esophageal sphincter into the esophagus, resulting in "heartburn".

"Heartburn" may also occur as a result of a weakening of the LES (Lower Esophageal Sphincter), because of overall liver energy deficit.

A weak LES valve allows stomach acid to leak through into the esophagus under "normal" stomach pressures. Western medicine calls this GERD (Gastro-Esophageal-Reflux-Disease) and will now recommend an anti-acid like Tums or Rolaids or even Pepsid or Nexium to relieve the pain from the chemical burn due to HCl in the esophagus.

If you reread the functions of HCl starting on page 75, you will be reminded that HCl is necessary to chelate minerals, which is necessary in order to get the minerals into the blood, which, in turn, are necessary to relax muscles and reduce spasms. It's also critical to drink fluids, especially if you're under stress for an extended period of time.

Spasms in any muscles in the body, including the smooth muscles in abdominal organs may result in sharp crampy pains, which most times can be resolved with the ingestion of water and minerals, especially magnesium citrate or some other form of magnesium (Magnesium Citrate is probably the most economical form of Magnesium. You can buy more effective forms, but they will be more expensive.) It's easy to become dehydrated, especially as we start to lose collagen as we age.

An old remedy that I recommend frequently for abdominal cramps and pain related to gall bladder and colon spasms also works well for any muscle spasm, including a stomach spasm due to emotional stress or low mineral concentration. To relieve a stomach or gall bladder spasm or in preparation for getting the stomach pulled out of the hole in the diaphragm, it would be advantageous to rub castor oil on the abdomen for two to three days prior, especially along the rib cage attachment of the abdominal muscle.

Put a towel or a rag over the oiled area and place a heating pad on it and sleep with it. If the all-night application is not practical, then at least use the heat with the castor oil application for a couple of hours while watching T.V. or working on the computer.

The castor oil will tend to relax the muscles of the diaphragm. The heat will drive the castor oil in to the muscles of the stomach to make it easier to pull it down or to "stretch" down by hanging. See the description and picture of the hanging procedure on page 118.

Another mechanical maneuver that I use frequently is the holding technique gleaned from Randolph Stone's teachings of Polarity. You can do this yourself, but it is much more effective if someone else does this for you.

If you're doing this for someone else, place all four fingers of your left hand on the abdominal muscle just under the rib cage of the person in front of you, and your right hand on the back immediately straight through the body from the position of your left hand. Just hold the position until you feel a "pulse" in your fingertips. You can actually feel the muscle of the stomach relax and release under the fingers of your left hand.

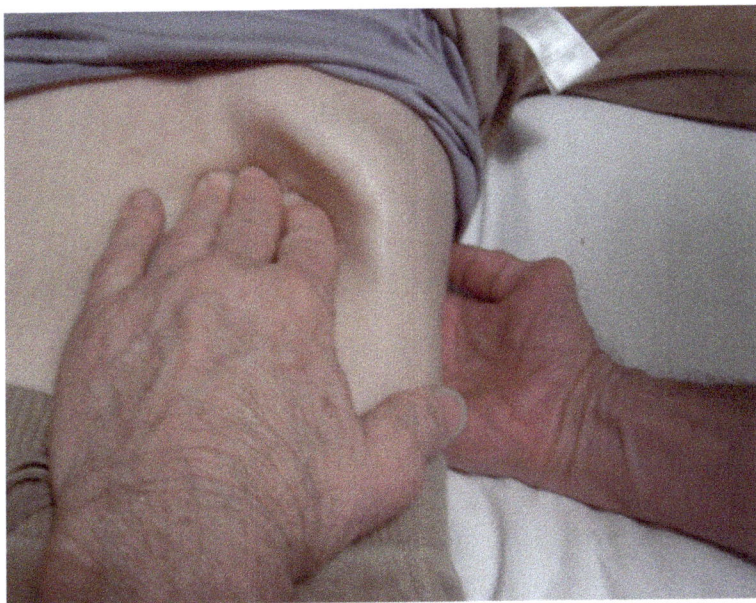

This technique can be used for a structural hiatal hernia as well as a functional hiatal hernia when the stomach is really "stuck" in the diaphragm. While maintaining a constant slight pressure on the stomach with your fingertips, you can "visualize" (see in your mind's eye) the stomach relaxing and moving downward. You may have to hold this position for a few minutes, but if you stay with it, you will feel it "let go". You can then with firm gentle pressure, stretch the stomach downward (towards the feet) away from the diaphragm.

I suggest that you reposition your hands to the position shown in the picture below.

CAUTION: See pages 104 & 105 before you attempt this move.

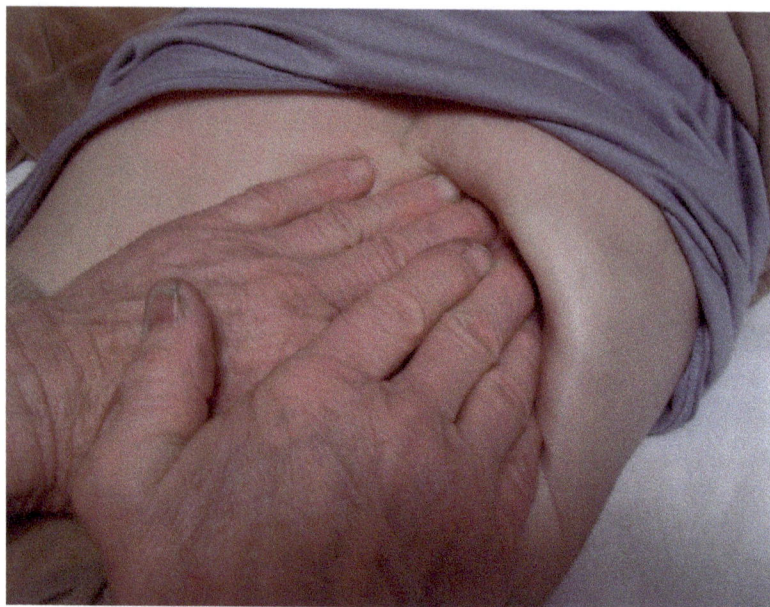

Again, this maneuver can be used for either a structural or a functional hiatal hernia. But for a structural hernia, you'll have to exert much more pulling pressure to get the stomach to slide out of the hiatus in the diaphragm, whereas, with a functional hiatal hernia, you only have to put gentle "holding" pressure on the stomach long enough to coax it to relax. Anxiety and emotional stress will cause the spasm in the stomach muscle that will affect the vagus nerve, resulting in all the symptoms of a classical Hiatal hernia syndrome that are listed above in the preceding pages.

The type of hiatal hernia that is commonly referred to as a **"sliding" hiatal hernia** is one in which the hiatus or hole in the diaphragm is rather loose and allows the stomach to "slide" in and out of the hole easily. This condition can in most cases be addressed with the holding technique with a little "tug" at the end. If it becomes stubborn, it can be coaxed down with the technique as shown in the picture above. Interestingly, this type of hiatal hernia will be the most difficult to deal with because of the stretched-out hole in the diaphragm.

The connective tissue that surrounds the hiatus in this case is very weak and will take more dedication and effort to strengthen it to keep the stomach down. The liver (in charge of the integrity of connective tissue) will need a lot of attention.

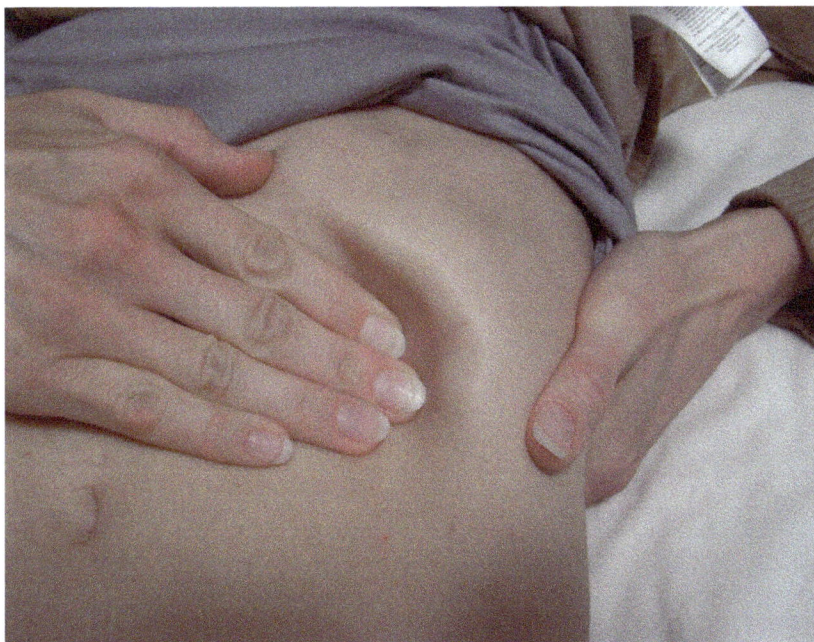

As mentioned, you can do this for yourself, in which case, you would place your right hand on the abdominal muscle on the left side of your body, just under the rib cage, and your left hand will slip under or onto your back immediately behind the point that your right hand is holding. It's best to be reclining for this maneuver so that you can relax your abdominal muscles easier.

If you are experiencing frequent stomach spasms and anxiety related digestive disturbances, it is best to eat nothing or very little, or food that digests quickly during periods of extreme stress, or drink water or other liquids, and then eat your bigger meal later after you can relax.

Most people do not realize that caffeine stimulates the adrenal glands, which is your "fight or flight juice". If you are under stress, caffeine will make your spasms worse.

And we must also keep in mind that the psoas muscle attaches to the diaphragm in the back, so that when the diaphragm is in trouble, the psoas muscle is affected.

Please keep in mind that the psoas muscle does in fact attach to the diaphragm as well as to the spine in the back and will be affected by the hernia condition. You will have to strengthen the psoas on both sides to stabilize the diaphragm.

The psoas muscle is the reserve tank muscle for the kidney, and if tight, will continue the injury to the diaphragm. Remember that caffeine in addition to stimulating the adrenal glands also puts a stress on the kidney, which affects the psoas muscle, which will draw energy from the diaphragm, which will result in the hernia symptom profile to continue.

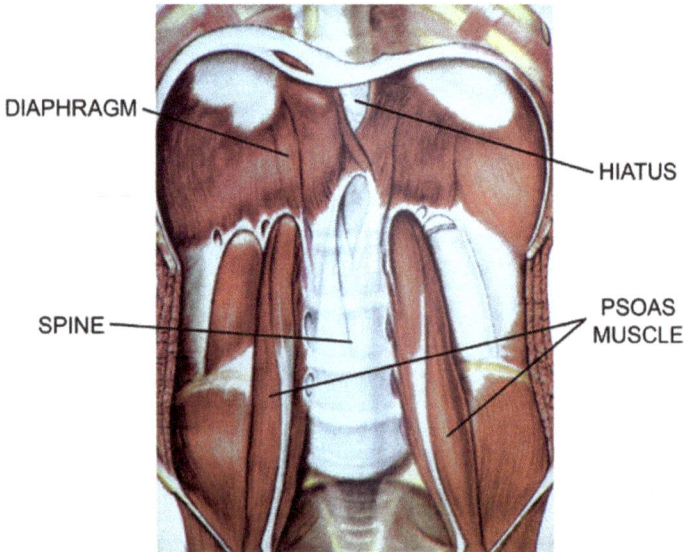

The upper trapezius muscle in the shoulders along with the psoas muscle in the low back is a "reserve tank" muscle for the kidneys. So you can expect back and shoulder pain and discomfort in the psoas AND upper trapezius muscles when the stomach and the diaphragm are irritated.

PHIL SELINSKY, N.D.

Pain in the back due to a psoas muscle contraction relating to kidney damage or stress, is covered in Volume II under "Back Pains". However, the Hiatal Hernia Syndrome is frequently the ultimate "bad guy" when dealing with mid back and shoulder pain because of the connection of the psoas muscle to the diaphragm. Pain creeps along and through connective tissue attachments.

Many folks will try to "stretch out" a spasm in a muscle. It's relatively easy to stretch a spasm out of a leg muscle or an arm muscle, or even a back muscle on occasion. But stretching a spasm out of a digestive tract muscle is more of a challenge. In addition, the related spasms in the diaphragm and psoas muscles are more difficult to stretch out. Therefore the holding technique described above will probably be your best move.

Remember the discussion on page 25, of a baby boy's bottom? That's exactly what the stomach does when you are under stress. If there is no physical damage to the hole in the diaphragm, the stomach will just "hug" the diaphragm for a while (functional hiatal hernia) resulting in the "temporary" symptoms of **hiatal hernia.**

If there is actual damage to the hole in the diaphragm, the stomach may many times scrunch itself up into the chest cavity (structural hiatal hernia) just from stress alone. This can put pressure against the heart resulting in palpitations. Pressure against the lungs will feel like some one is sitting on your chest when you try to breathe. You may also feel a tightness or constriction or cramping pain all around the bottom of the rib cage and down the mid back where the diaphragm attaches to the psoas muscle.

This is the situation (structural hiatal hernia) that can actually be seen on an x-ray or a scan. Western medicine's answer to this is anti acids. And if that doesn't do the job, there is always surgery. As I have stated in Volume II, surgery is rather final. Once you've cut something off or out, you cannot put it back later after you found out that the procedure did not work. All of these listed symptoms are instantly relieved as soon as the stomach is pulled "out of the hole". One of the immediate tests is to take a deep breath.

There will be more room in the chest cavity. You will be able to breath easier. The palpitations will be gone. The "lump in your throat" will be gone. If any of these symptoms persist, you didn't get the stomach all the way out. You'll have to try again.

If you have an actual structural hiatal hernia with part of the stomach above the diaphragm, as in the picture on page 24, the ONLY answer is to have someone pull the stomach down out of the hole for you and then religiously follow the suggestions listed below for at least one to two years to allow the hernia in the diaphragm to heal.

Of course the healing time will be dependant on how you care for the liver, since the liver energy is responsible for the integrity of connective tissue in the body. (See Volume II)

If you are experiencing a **<u>functional</u> hiatal hernia** (from stress) as opposed to a **<u>structural</u> hiatal hernia** (an actual tear in the diaphragm), you could try the suggestions listed above first. But if the stress that is causing your functional hiatal hernia symptoms is overwhelming, you might still need to actually pull the stomach down to stretch it out. Some spasms are stubborn.

Sometimes when you experience a muscle spasm, stretching the muscle will "pull" the spasm out. The stomach IS a muscle and can also spasm and create all the symptoms of the classic **hiatal hernia syndrome** in which case, "pulling the spasm out" will relax the stomach and take the pressure and stress off of the vagus nerve so that the symptoms disappear immediately.

I realize that this creates a challenging situation for most people because allopathic medical doctors are NOT taught to "touch" the body. They have been trained to do their diagnosing from a distance, using drugs and surgery to solve all the problems presented to them. As the story unfolds in Volume I, in order to solve a seemingly impossible problem, sometimes you have to journey "outside the box" for the answer to the problem.

Chiropractors are trained to "touch" the body, but they do not get much if any training in visceral (gut) manipulation.

Osteopaths were at one time trained exclusively to manipulate bone and connective tissue including visceral organs and cranial bones. But they sold out to the Morris Fishbein (AMA) crowd and are almost exclusively involved in pharmaceuticals (drugs) now. So that leaves a few of us old relics who still believe that physical manipulation can help this human machine to achieve homeostasis.

Connective Tissue has a Memory

After the stomach is pulled out of the hole in the diaphragm, **YOU** must keep it there. There is a tendency for connective tissue to behave just like Silly Putty. It has a memory. When you stretch it, it wants to go back to its former shape.

Therefore it may take a few encounters of pulling the stomach down before it "learns" to stay where you put it.

In addition, any pressure on the abdomen will cause the stomach to want to crawl back up into the diaphragm where it has been living for a considerable length of time. For most people, it has been there all their lives.

As you get older, you start to feel the discomfort more acutely and are finally motivated to do something about it. Remember that you were born with a genetic weakness in the liver energy circuit, which resulted in the weak muscle and connective tissue that developed into a hernia.

This is the hardest part of all for you to remember to do to keep the stomach out of the hole in the diaphragm:

No bending over from the waist.
No tight clothing around the middle.
No sit-ups.
No crunches.
No up-side-down positions.
No yoga positions that emphasize headstands or bending at the waist.

As soon as you wake up in the morning, drink a glass of water (If you have reflux add one tablespoon of apple cider vinegar to the water) and then get up on your tippy toes and drop forcefully back on your heels. The water puts weight in the stomach and jumping back on your heels causes gravity and inertia to "hammer" the stomach back down where it belongs.

AND MOST IMPORTANT OF ALL - HANG ... HANG ... HANG

As often throughout the day as you can, find some place to hang. (See pictures)

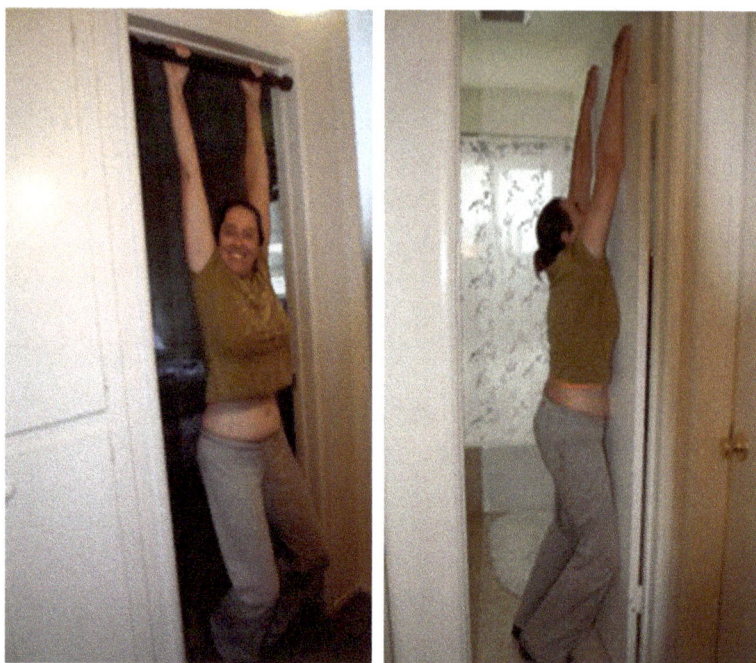

You can build a bar in a doorway or hang on a door (if you do hang on a door, hang close to the hinges so you don't end up with the door on the floor on top of you.).

You can hang on a car door or anything that is handy. You can even lean up against the wall with your hands above your head. You do not have to have your feet off the floor. You are not doing chin-ups.

Just hold on to something with your hands and let your whole body become loose. It's a stretch. Hang for about 10 seconds each time. But you want to hang as often as you can remember. Paste signs all over your house or office ... "**HANG**".

The body weight pulls against your shoulders, which lifts your rib cage, which flattens the diaphragm, which allows the stomach to drop down where it belongs.

In our earlier conversation, I mentioned that, if you are experiencing a **"functional hiatal hernia"** episode, hanging will usually relieve the symptoms. This means that if the stomach is just scrunched up against the diaphragm and not protruding through the diaphragm, you can do this to stretch it out and relieve the telltale symptoms.

Sometimes though it may actually need to be "pulled". It depends on the severity of the stress in the moment and the tenacity of your connective tissue.

The objective here is to keep the stomach down and away from the diaphragm for a long enough time to let the damaged tissue heal. This can take anywhere from 6 months to 2 years, depending on your age and behavior. If the stomach goes back up again, the clock starts all over again.

Once the overstretched hole in the diaphragm has closed and healed, you can return to somewhat of a "normal" life again. But, you have to keep in mind that the integrity of your connective tissue is a genetic issue and is closely related to the liver energy stress.

So if you continue to "sin" with nicotine, caffeine, alcohol, refined sugar, refined flour, dairy products, and drugs, along with improper food combining and extreme stress, you will probably have a real tough time overcoming the problem with the overwhelmed liver energy and the resulting stomach damage (from the hernia) or any dis – ease condition in the body for that matter.

> *REMEMBER THAT "NATURE" IS ALWAYS IN BALANCE ... IF YOU PUT "NATURE" OUT OF BALANCE (with your behavior) "NATURE" WILL RETURN TO BALANCE ... OFTEN WITH A VENGENCE AND TO YOUR INDIVIDUAL DETRIMENT.*

Bioflex – Meditech Laser Treatment

In my practice, I also use the Meditec Bioflex Low Intensity Laser device to "soften" the diaphragm muscle before attempting to pull the stomach down. This is in addition to the castor oil packs a week or so before trying to pull a "stubborn" (spasming) stomach. Usually the stomach will slide out of the hole with a minimum of effort. But there are always the exceptions that resist the easy way.

In addition, I use the Bioflex device after the "pull" to encourage the healing process of the stomach and the herniated hiatus (stretched hole) in the diaphragm.

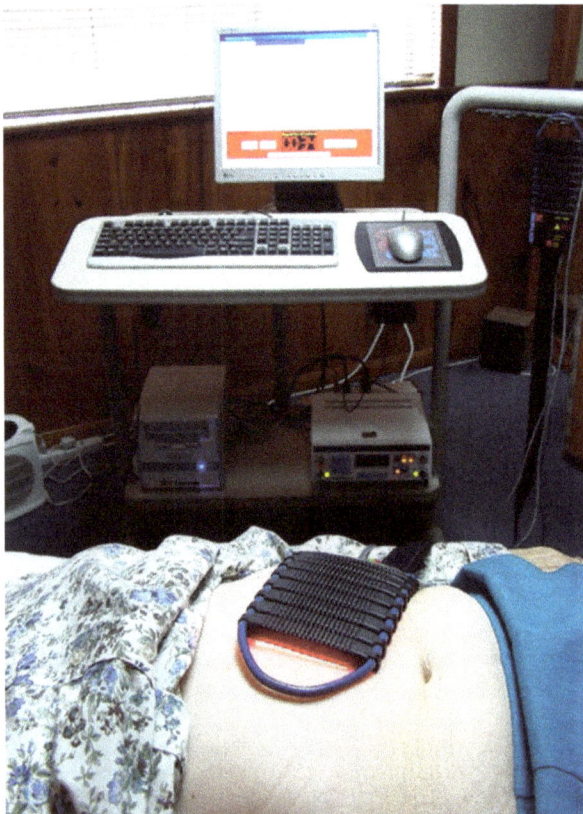

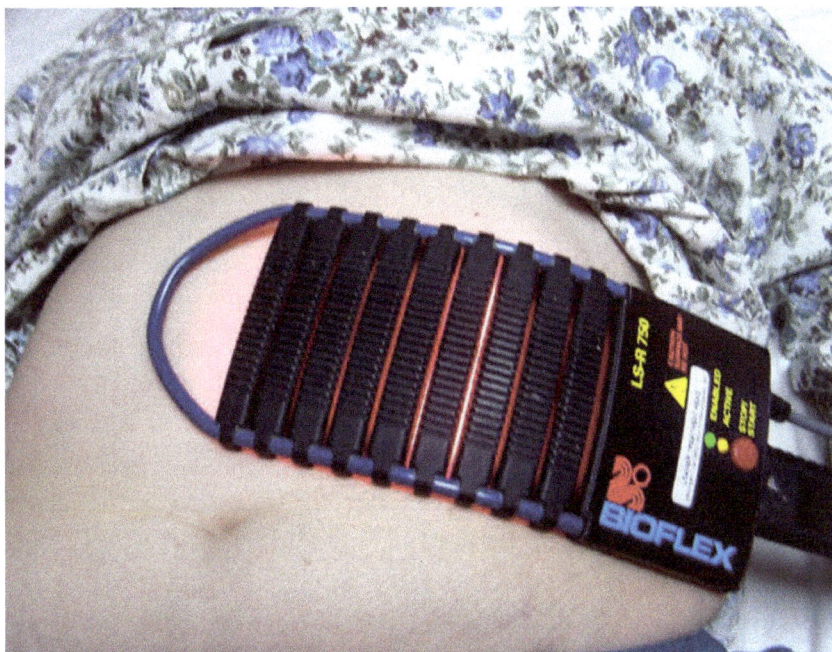

The Bioflex apparatus uses photon (packets of light) energy to encourage the healing process. First, the L.E.D. pad delivers incoherent (no specific direction) red light, then infra red light, then the coherent (lined up light waves) red LASER light to the damaged tissues.

Check out their web site <http://www.bioflexlaser.com> for a practitioner in your area that might use this device. This is a very useful tool for sports injuries and healing after surgeries like hip and knee replacements. It also has been used successfully on open lesions and necrosing tissue from advanced diabetes.

Meditech also produces the "home use" version of this device, which is much less expensive than the professional model, and it is very portable and easy to use.

Fred Kahn, M.D., one of the foremost experts in the field of cold laser applications for damaged tissue, directs the clinical operation at the home office in Toronto, Canada.

Toll free # 888-557-4004   Tel: (416) 251-1055
Email: info@bioflexlaser.com

Royal Raymond Rife's Beam Ray Device

Back in the 1920's and 30's, Royal Raymond Rife discovered that everything has a "mortal oscillating rate" … a frequency vibration at which any entity will actually literally blow up or fragment. A crystal will shatter if it is subjected to a certain sound frequency. A popular example is that of a singer's voice reaching a specific pitch that will shatter a wine glass.

Rife discovered that germs and viruses have certain specific "mortal oscillating rates" that if subjected to that frequency from a frequency generator can be killed … shattered … exploded. He built a device that would broadcast a radio frequency that would kill germs and viruses associated with certain diseases. Because of his tremendous success, he was persecuted and prosecuted by the established medical community headed by a Morris Fishbein, M.D. The "powers that be" were fearful that their entire industry that was centered around pharmaceuticals and surgery would be destroyed if this concept of controlling disease with resonance were to "catch on". Unfortunately, money trumps ethics.

A number of people over the years have attempted to duplicate the device from salvaged lab notes and first hand memories of lab technicians. There are numerous technical issues that have prevented the exact duplication of Rife's device … until now.

Mr. Lynn Kenny from Alabama has succeeded in creating a "Beam Ray" device that has been shown to do everything that the original Rife frequency generator could do plus reducing and/or eliminating pain associated with serious debilitating and degenerative conditions.

I have had first hand experience with the Beam Ray. "It was a dark and stormy night …" Seriously, It was dark in my living room late at night and I tripped over a coffee table and put my hand out to catch myself from falling onto the table. Unbeknownst to me, the family cat decided to spend the night on the table and my hand landed on the cat. Naturally, he was surprised at this "attack" and he bit me on the wrist. One puncture wound was deep and was bleeding so I put Yunnan Payao (a Chinese herbal remedy for gun-shot wounds) on it and the other wound looked to be just skin deep, so I did not put anything on it. By morning, the cat tooth wound with the Yunnan Payao on it looked like it was just fine. However, the one that I did not treat looked infected. I put Yunnan Payao on the infected wound, but it was too late. It got worse. By the next day my hand and wrist was swollen to twice its normal size and I was feverish and shaky. There was a red line observable moving up my forearm almost to my elbow. I thought, "Hmmmmm, I think I'm in trouble".

A client-friend of mine had just purchased a Beam Ray device to treat her cat that had cancer. So I thought what have I got to lose. I sat under the Beam Ray for about 1½ hours and by morning the infection was gone. The swelling was gone. The red line was gone. The pain was gone. The wound took about a week to heal, but the infection was totally gone the first night.

I have since seen that the Beam Ray device has also successfully obliterated candida in many of my patients that have used the Beam Ray upon my recommendation. Systemic Candida is very difficult to kill. Once it gets into the blood, it takes months and in some cases years of serious effort to get rid of it. The Beam Ray also seems to be able to assist body tissue to build and repair itself.

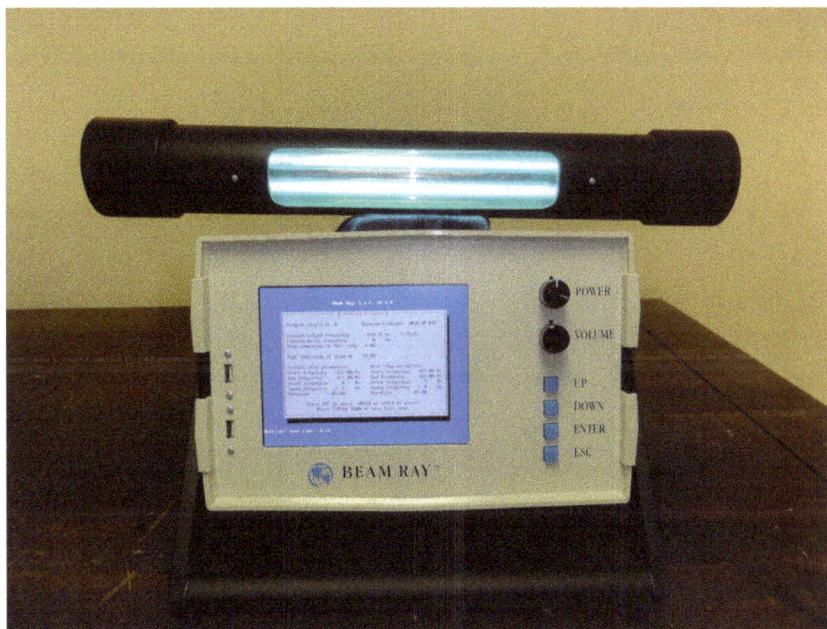

Any questions and/or information about the Beam Ray can be addressed to:
(205) 543-6356
FAX: (205) 543-6357
e-mail: <support@ft-beamray.com>
Direct e-mail: <ftbeamray@gmail.com>
Facebook: facebook.com/THEbeamray

I would like to reemphasize at this point that it's the weakness in the liver circuit that results in the hernia in the diaphragm that damages the stomach that leads to putrefaction of the food.

As the food rots in your intestines, it contaminates the blood and lymph system. The liver has to work overtime to remove the toxins from the blood and consequently has less energy to maintain integrity of the connective tissue in the body, especially the diaphragm, which exacerbates the hernia situation.

(Reread the Series Circuit concept on page 45 and the Motor Home Model on page 52.)

It is therefore imperative that we "clean house" to take the stress off of the immune system. We can do this by improving the rate and efficiency of the fluid distribution system in the body.

Exercise, deep breathing, muscle massage and acupuncture point and reflex point stimulation will help to clean the blood so that stress can be removed from the liver so that the connective tissue can heal.

I have created a DVD set that takes the viewer through a full body scanning and treatment procedure. In the DVD, I explain the location and function of the major pressure points and organ reflex relationships between muscles and organ function and integrity.

I show a systematic procedure to determine the source of aches and pains and what can be done to alleviate most chronic pains and degenerative conditions. If you check YouTube for my name "Phil Selinsky, N.D.", I have posted a video titled: FULL BODY REFLEX ROUTINE TRAILER. To obtain this DVD set, please refer to my web site <thehumanmachine.com> for purchase instructions, or send an e-mail request to <ihss@earthlink.net>.

Also check my web site for the dates and locations of the latest seminars and classes.

In closing, I would like to emphasize this concept:

Live what you believe and believe what you live ...
Your kids and grandkids are watching you.

Challenge

I have yet to see an individual with a cancer problem who DID NOT also first have a problem with HCl concentration in the stomach from either a functional disturbance or a structural abnormality or both, and a corresponding difficulty with blood contamination from the large intestine.

This is a formal and official request for anyone to prove me wrong. Show me a case of cancer cell growth anywhere in the body that was NOT preceded by an HCl inhibition. This of course exempts but does not exclude situations involving traumatic and chronic tissue damage from chemicals and/or radiation.

Critical Note

As mentioned earlier in this text, each organ in the body has an energy function, which includes emotions. Extreme emotional pressure, whether internalized or openly expressed, can affect the integrity and health of the physical organ that is associated with the emotion.

Caustic stress can cause physical damage to organs, which result in any one or all of the symptom profiles discussed in this book series.

Intense

Fear affects the kidneys and bladder

Anger and **resentment** affects the liver and gall bladder

Shocking disappointment affects the heart, small intestine, circulation, and thyroid/adrenals

Lack of **joy** and or **purpose** affects the stomach and pancreas

Grief affects the large intestine and lungs.

And remember that chronic pain and discomfort in the "reserve tank" muscles can signal "trouble in River City" with the organ(s) related to them. Study the Ache and Pain Profiles in Volume II of this series and pay attention to the "dash board gages" on your "HUMAN MACHINE".

Please stay in touch with me regarding the availability dates of classes, seminars, and private counseling sessions through my web site <thehumanmachine. com> or e-mail <ihss@earthlink.net>.

APPENDIX I

TESTIMONIALS

Please note: These testimonials were copied directly from the original e-mails that were sent to me. I only changed some punctuation and a few grammatical errors. Otherwise they are exactly as presented to me. - Thank you -

"I have known Phil Selinsky for over 25 years, and a person more dedicated and qualified to discuss the workings of the living body would be hard to find. In his excellent new book, **THE HUMAN MACHINE: A Trouble Shooter's Manual Volume III**, Phil has managed to turn what could be a dry, technical subject into an exciting, interesting page-turner sure to enthuse and inform both professional and lay person alike."
- *Harvey Diamond*, N.Y. Times Bestselling author, **FIT FOR LIFE** -

The Human Machine, Hiatal Hernia Syndrome Epidemic, is a book about a complicated subject made easy by the brilliant words of Dr. Phil. His understanding of anatomy and physiology have made him a pioneer in the treatment and healing of the human body. Thousands of his patients have benefited by his hands and recommendations. Dr. Phil's non-surgical treatments have saved patients great expense and suffering. His book gives a healthy, unconventional treatment that includes easy to understand and perform self help advice. This is a masterpiece for anyone who is responsible for his own health and healing. Thank you Dr. Phil!
- *Artista J. Marchioni, RN, BSN, LE, CLNC, HHP* -

I have known Dr. Phil since 2003. I am very thankful and take comfort in all his naturopathic teachings in many areas of my health. He has taught me a more realistic approach in my health problems and that you learn that your body really is your temple. You must begin to care for it and treat

it with respect. He taught me how to manage my condition and improve my health by taking daily digestive enzymes, how to combine my foods, juicing, and many good herbal meds instead of taking over-the-counter meds and has taught me a whole new arsenal of treatments and insights about many health issues. I feel I am in a much better area with my health with his expertise and direction and I am very thankful and appreciative for his advice and I now design my life to live as healthy as I can.
- *Rose Patrick* –

May I say the following about your care of my body?
After being diagnosed with Prostate Cancer, my daughter, Cyndi and her husband Doug suggested I see Dr. Phil Selinsky, ND, for another option to surgery. After our first meeting and discussion of what I would have to do to make this option work, I Prayed for direction from our LORD JESUS CHRIST as it would require a change in my eating habits. This was not the top thing on my list of things to do. I enjoyed eating all the great foods that man has doctored up to taste great ... chips and cheese, pork, donuts, chocolate and on goes the list. My thought was if GOD would help me stay on the diet Dr. Phil wanted me on, then I would do it. I have, with HIS help, eaten nothing but what Dr. Phil approved for the passed 3 years and it was not that hard. My daughter really was a great help to start with and I would not have been able to do this if it were not for her preparing a salad of vegetables every week for those first few months. Now I'm doing it and my LORD continues to bless these things to bring me better health. Three years ago I was a bit overweight, if you would have asked me, but no big deal, as I'm 6 foot 3 inch and weighed 230. I eat like a horse never was hungry, the salads were without dressings of any kind, but I eat my fill every meal. Within 6 months I was down to 190 and the lowest I got to was 176 and then put back about 10 pounds and now weigh between 185 and 190 for the past couple of years and the body is working much better, but what of the Prostate. My PSA score in the beginning was 10.6 and dropped to a low of 7.6 November, 2011 and three weeks ago was at 8.0. None of this would have happened without the help of Dr. Phil. The world has a Doctor Phil and so do I, but his last name is Selinsky. No, I have not forgotten the LORD, for without JESUS there would be not Dr.

Phil and soon there would have been no Fred. Oh, yes, the Medical Doctor says "Good job, Fred.

We keep an eye on the rest of the body with tests." Thank you Doctor Phil Selinsky and GOD BLESS you and your family and patients.
- *Fred Boettcher*, **Boettcher Engineering & Contracting** -

Dr. Phil is a healer who cares about his patients and who tells us the truth. And heals too. Thank you, Phil Selinsky."
- *Peter Eastman*, L.L.D. -

When I first met Dr. Phil, I had a headache every day, I had heartburn after I ate anything. I had a low back pain and neck pain that would make me lie down and take pain killers like candy. My knees ached so bad I could not step off of a curb without stinging pain. I went to the emergency room many times for what I thought was a heart attack, but it wasn't. I had a difficult time leaving the house, because of fear of crowds. I drove my friends and family away with anger and violent behavior. The whites of my eyes were always bright red, which made dealing with the police somewhat of an adventure. They insisted that I walk the white line on the side of the road because they were convinced that I had to be drunk or high on drugs or something. I had been to medical doctors since I was 11 years old looking for the answers for my troubles. When Dr. Phil said that he was willing to help me, I was incredulous. I am pretty sure that I yelled and threatened him. He worked on me anyway. He said that I had to make some changes in my diet and I would be better. He laid out a program for me to follow for what he called "hiatal hernia syndrome". Within 4 months most of my complaints were gone. That was May of 1994. I will always remember that that was the day that I started to get better. It has been 18 years of no headaches, no back pain, no knee pain, no violent behavior, no red eyes, and a peace of mind that I never had through most of my life. I will always be thankful for Phil's never giving up on me.
- *Carl Coffee, HHP* -

Anyone suffering without relief, who has tried all other avenues for pain relief and is still looking for the underlying problem, should read this book by Dr. Phil Selinsky. After years of searching for answers, I finally found

Dr. Phil. He has solved many "mysteries" of what it takes to heal the body and live a meaningful life.
- *Barbara Rogers Scollin, C.P.A.* -

Dr. Phil, you and the application of your philosophy of the The Human Machine has greatly affected my life. In working with you, and you working on my "machine" over these years; I have instituted certain approaches in selfcare. Regularly, I feed my cells complimentary fuel via astragalus, killer T-Cell regulation, exercise, protein, hydration, balanced cell symbiosis, regular massage and tune-ups with your touch and corrective positioning of my body's inner software and hardware (organs and musculoskeletal). I utilized this approach during my recovery from a near death experience as a result of a 2008 helicopter crash. My Level 1 injuries were such that I incurred 43 fractures including the lower back and shattered right femur, traumatic and intense brain injury, potential loss of an eye, partial amputation, major muscle loss, 40% third degree burns on lower extremities requiring extensive skin grafts and internal organ loss. I was unable to walk for approx. 1 1/2 years, walk with assistance for another year and can now walk unassisted with orthotics and shoes. Without shoes I still require a wheelchair. I received approximately 30 surgeries within a few years span. Because of my blessed mental and physical approach to my recovery, coupled with fantastic medical care, including yours, I have had a miraculous recovery. To look at me today; one would not ascertain from external appearance the multitudinous transgressions that occurred to "my" Human Machine. Thank you for sharing your philosophy and mechanical administrations with me over these years. They are integrated into my personal philosophy and approach, dramatically effecting and improving my life every day.
With love and respect, - *Laura Sharpe* -

"Many moons ago, (33+ years) I experienced much pain in my body and had a problem walking. A friend recommended Dr. Phil and I made an appointment. He helped me a lot as a Dr of Holistic Medicine and recognized the imbalance of my body electrical circuits. His techniques for relief of a hiatal hernia brought permanent relief! I was so grateful. I became a student of his and learned much more. Prior to this, I was

working in the medical field and did not receive relief of symptoms. I am eternally grateful for his assistance, his teaching, and his friendship for these many years! His teaching and experience are invaluable. His books are precise and clear! His devotion to helping others heal is rare! I followed his techniques for many years with great success and am now retired.
- MB -

I have known Dr. Phil Selinsky for ten years and He totally changed my health and the way I look at physical illness. I started to have low back pain since I was about 11 years old. Standing still or sitting with straight back is unbearable for me. Before I met Dr. Phil, I went to see many Western doctors and Chinese traditional doctors. None of them has helped me. They don't even know why I had pain. When I first see Dr. Phil, He explained that what was wrong and why it was wrong with the body I live in. What he told me was totally mind blowing. Now I am living pain free. Thanks Dr. Phil! For the past 10 years, I only see my family doctor for annual physical only. If there is any discomfort for the body, I'll go to see Phil and will feel like new person next day without side effect (drugs). Once again thank you Phil!
- Helen Castner -

I was a patient of Dr. Phil Selinsky in the past, then I moved away and saw other Naturopathic doctors. I couldn't wait to move back so I could be taken care of by Dr. Phil once more. He knows the human body inside and out like no other. His care, recommendations and valuable information have been and will continue to be life changing for me.
- Susan Richardson -

I have always known there was a better way to care for my health. With some help I found Dr. Phil. (I have excellent medical insurance, but have chosen the holistic approach. All of the following conditions have been diagnosed and treated by western medical procedures. Some have been helpful, others harmful; and pharmaceuticals, some helpful, some do nothing, but all have harmful side effects).

I am a 64 year old male diagnosed with the following medical conditions. Along with the medical diagnosis are Dr. Phil's suggestions to mitigate the symptoms:

1. Manic/Depressive. Homeopathic preparations and a variety of natural herbs have been helpful. Yoga and meditation work wonders. (Phil has also recommended an excellent Homeopathic Dr. for further consultation for this and other problems if and when necessary.)
2. Insomnia. Several herbs and homeopathic remedies along with meditation and mindfulness have helped.
3. Hiatel Hernia resulting in GERD. Phil repositioned my stomach, told me not to bend over, and I hang form a bar several times a day.

The condition is much improved, but will take time to completely heal.

4. Medial Epicondilitis (golfer's elbow). Collagen and Silica supplements, Crystal therapy, Physical Therapy ... Pain is gone.
5. Arthritis. Hyaluronic acid fixed the knees. No more Ace bandages. I can play golf, kayak, and bike without pain.
6. Benign Prostate Hyperplasia. Flower Pollen, and Histidine.
7. Diabetes. Lost 25lbs, and changed diet. No more need for Metformin.
8. High blood pressure & high cholesterol. Same as #7 ... No more pills.

All of the above can and will be cured with a proper diet and proper food combining. This is easier said than done, but I am working on it. The full body Reflexology Massage Dr. Phil gives me weekly keeps me tuned up. He can tell me things (just by touch) about my body that I would otherwise have no knowledge of. I have been seeing Dr. Phil since March 2009, and will continue to see him as long as he continues to work. His teachings have been invaluable in my effort to lead a more healthy life. Dr. Phil is a wealth of information; psychological, life experience, as well as suggestions for physical changes.

- John Knudsen, R.N. -

Term of Treatment: April 2011 to present date

* Outstanding results with physical manipulation of stomach area.. to return the stomach to its natural position, and thereby reduce GERD like symptoms
* Similiar results with Hiatal Hernia problems--gained many ideas on tips to maintain the positive results from sessions (ie: hang)
* Sessions produce a wealth of positive relaxation feelings; reduction of pain in all areas, but especially my targeted problems (stomach, lower intestinal areas)
* Use of the laser technology also beneficial to increase comfort and reduce pain of lower gut.
* Dr Phil has been a tremendous resource for natural remedies and options that assist the body to do what it needs (lower blood pressure).
* All sessions have been educative and positive!
* Truly almost a year of learning about how our bodies function and respond to correct stimuli and lifestyle changes to better support natural bodily functions.
* Many referrals have been given that utilize different practitioners and techniques...healing codes; Rife beam ray; Chinese herbs. This reflects a true interest in assisting and educating, not just making money from a client and keeping the client for his own practice.

- Stephen Phelps -

Wow, where do I begin with my testimonies of 30 years of being a client of Dr. Phil. From body tune-ups to urgent-care visits he has always discovered the "hidden imbalances" that the western clinicians miss. I received Dr. Phil's body treatments, follow-up advice and supplement recommendations after a recent appendectomy. Phil discovered my health was in jeopardy with a compromised digestive system, a weakened liver, intestinal blocks and lurking appendix parasites. There was not one medical test while in the hospital that could determine any of this or the hiatal hernia Dr. Phil was most concerned about. His recommendation of betaine hydrochoride & slippery elm began to turn things around for me.

Dr. Phil Selinsky saved my life and got my entire system on track to "optimum health". He is a true master "body mechanic".
- **Candice Wilson** – Facials of Essence, Ojai

I have known Phil Selinsky for over 20 years. He has helped me, my family, and many of my friends over the years through his wisdom and knowledge of the human body. What I especially appreciate about Phil is that he works with you as a whole person. What I mean by that is he not only has the knowledge of how the organs, muscles, bones, etc. work. But he also works with your emotions, meridians, massage, trigger points, your eating habits, and many other modalities. Whatever it takes to get you better. His knowledge is so vast, and he never ceases to amaze me. I am so excited that he's writing this book. I have so many testimonials of how Phil has helped, but I will just name a few:

1. In 2000 I was diagnosed with 3rd stage melanoma on my hip. Western medicine gave me 6 months to live. I contacted Phil, he said to use compound X. It was gone within about 5 months. I never had any chemotherapy, nor did I have any radiation. It has been 11 years and there isn't a trace of any cancer in my body.

2. My sister had pneumonia, the doctors put her on antibiotics. After about 2 weeks she wasn't getting any better. So I called Phil. He said get her Whole leaf aloe liquid. Within 2 days she was feeling better.

3. My sister had been hit by a car as a pedestrian in her 20's and for 10 years she had suffered with pain in her body. One night she called me because she couldn't lift her neck. I called Phil. He came right over to her house and worked on her. After just 2 sessions, she was pain free and could move her neck. Phil said her body was holding on to fear.

4. My 18 year old son was living in a place where he got sick with a lung infection. He was coughing, spitting up colored flem, had no energy, and his skin was pale. This went on for about 3 months. Finally he let me call Phil for help. Phil said get Olive leaf extract and Cat's claw. Within 2 or 3 days he was on the road to recovery.

5. Another time I called Phil because I had run a fever of 102 to 104 for 4 days. I was in and out of consciousness and hallucinating. Phil asked me to look down my throat and tell me if it was white? It was. he said you have Strep throat and to get the Cat's claw and Olive leaf extract. Within hours I was better, no more fever.

Again I'm so glad Phil is putting out this book to help people and give them a choice over Western medicine . I appreciate having alternatives. If not for Phil and his knowledge of Compound X, I would not be here today.
- *Melody Mewbourne* - Thousand Oaks CA

Thanks for the chance to express my gratitude for teaching me to better understand the function of my body. Most of all when it speaks to me through pain or symptoms. For this I have little need or use for Western Medical Doctors. Your knowledge and teachings have helped me to find natural ways to improve my health and wellbeing. My life has changed and improved from your help. I will be forever grateful.
- *Michelle V.* -

I have known Dr. Phil Selinsky for the past 25 years. Dr. Phil is a "Master Mechanic of the Body". His knowledge and expertise have helped me in ways too numerous to mention. When I met Phil 25 years ago, western medicine wanted to remove my gallbladder. Thanks to Dr. Phil, I still have my gallbladder to this day.

He has helped me over come the devastating effects of Candida, Celiac Disease, Leaky Gut Syndrome and a traumatic fall this past Christmas. My daughter Danika and I have also benefited from his Hiatal Hernia protocol. His Reflexology routine has been the best healing tool I have ever encountered. I am most grateful to Dr. Phil and am convinced that I would not be alive today had it not been for him and his vast wealth of wisdom and knowledge.
- *Dianne McCown, LVN, HHP* -

It's hard to sum up quickly everything I want to say. I want to speak to how you always educate me and get me thinking about life changes for the better, to speak about how much you clearly love your work... to speak

about how caring you are of your clients, etc... but it would be too long. I am an endurance athlete with a stressful job, which is very demanding on my body. To maintain my health and to bring me back into balance, I have regular appointments with Dr. Phil Selinksy. After a session with Dr. Selinsky, I feel stronger, energized, clear, balanced and grounded. My digestion has improved. My ability to handle stress has improved. My running has improved. Thank you Dr. Phil.
- P.W. -

Dr. Phil treated my hiatal hernia by pulling the stomach down into place. His treatment to heal the organs in my stomach was successful and my intestines, liver, kidney etc. are functioning perfectly now. This means that my health is excellent. A recent sigmoidoscopy caused the MD to exclaim about how healthy my colon looked - clean (no polyps) strong, and beautiful. I attribute that to the treatments I have received from Dr. Phil.
- Harriet S. -

One visit to Dr. Phil Selinsky changed my life. After he adjusted my hiatal hernia, I could breath more deeply than I had been able to in years! I consequently have more energy and better digestion. After several visits, I noticed my IBS had subsided considerably. Dr. Phil is truly a gifted healer, treating patients with brilliant skill and genuine caring. He is also a wealth of valuable information and teaches easy and effective self-care techniques.
- Madelyn Reusser -

I first went to Dr. Phil with a severe digestion problem with acid reflux and trouble with bowel movements. He assessed that situation and found my stomach way up under my ribs. He made an adjustment and told me what to do to keep it down where it belongs. He also made what I considered a radical change in my diet. After all I was the Pasta Queen with lots of cheese. After sticking to the diet mostly for a few weeks all my reflux troubles vanished and I have not had them since. Dr. Phil is a genius at diagnosing a problem and fixing it with reflexive manipulation and energy work. He also referred me to various other specialists over the years and has suggested trying various supplements. I invariably learn something new on each visit and am gradually fixing long time genetic problems. As a result,

I am in better health than I was twenty years ago and continue to improve. When I had to cut back on expenses due to retirement, I said that I would give up lots of other things but not my visits with Phil.
- *Dr. Gina Shaw* -

My treatment history with Dr. Phil Selinsky has spanned over 3 decades. I first came to him as a student back in 1981. I graduated from his year-long course with my Holistic Health Practitioner's certificate. He said to me upon one of my first treatments with him "If you keep on eating and drinking like you are now, your liver will take you out". He told me I was born with a weak liver circuit due to alcoholism in my family history. I of course stopped everything that was detrimental to my health and embraced a whole new healthy life style...NOT! I continued to assault my liver with an assortment of sugar, alcohol, caffeine, chemicals, processed and refined foods, dairy, and so on. Over the years I would show up at Phil's door with a sore lower back or some malady that was easily remedied and then I would be on my way again. In 2002, I came to Dr. Phil with a horrendous pain in the arse. It was my sciatic nerve acting up. I could not sit, stand, lie down, or walk without excruciating pain. I received 5 treatments over a period of 2 weeks and at the end of the fifth treatment he said, "You have something growing inside you. I want you to go to the ER and have a CT scan from the sternum to the pubic bone". I did just that and the ER doctor informed me that there was a 6-centimeter tumor in my liver as well as a smaller one and that it appeared to have metastasized to the bone in my spine.

That is when I finally woke up and decided to give my lifestyle a complete overhaul. That was 10 years ago and since no longer ingesting any acid producing substances, I feel as though I have cheated time. I feel and look better than I have in at least 20 years. I have absolutely zero joint pain and that was my biggest complaint up till about 8 years ago. I can run and do aerobic exercise classes like I did in my twenties. In case you are not doing the math, I am now 55 years young. I know without Dr. Phil's expertise my tumors would have gone unnoticed till it was way too late and I would not have been given the jolt I needed to pave the way to a whole new world,

both physically, psychologically, and emotionally. With great love and great respect I am honored to share my experiences.
Thank you. *- Kate Danta, LVN, HHP -*

Dr. Phil is truly a great healer. He is famous for his six-day-per- week, early-morning to late night schedule with clients, and he has been following that schedule for over four decades. With this vast, clinical experience, a keen intellect and his engineering background, Phil has discovered his own, unique approach to healing the Human Machine. Using his uncanny ability to correctly diagnose, and using often self-discovered, but always effective and gentle treatments,

Phil tells clients what has gone wrong and shows them the path back to good health. Dr. Phil's work on hiatal hernia is groundbreaking. He not only has identified the overlooked epidemic in our midst, but he also has shown how to gently diagnose the syndrome and how to restore full health.
- Keith Milliken, PhD. - Grangeville, Idaho

Dr. Selinsky is a master mechanic of the human machine. It may seem to his patients that "Dr. Phil" has an uncanny ability to "read" the body, but he will tell you it is just plain science, because he understands it inside and out. He hears our complaints: the pain in the shoulder, the dry mouth at night, an unusual stomach ache, etc., and readily interprets these symptoms as clues to what the body is lacking in terms of nutrition, or suffering from through overindulgence, or responding to in terms of injury or accident. Dr. Phil bases all of his analysis on a thorough knowledge of how the body actually operates, and how it naturally responds to environment, diet and injury.

It is a fascinating lesson in anatomy and nutrition when Phil explains precisely how the body works and what is happening. Moreover it is a relief to understand and empowering to know how to be in control of your health. I would expect Dr. Selinsky's new book will bring to readers what patients have appreciated learning from him.
- E.T. Garcia -

Dr. Phil has an extraordinary understanding and ability to get to the causal level of stomach stress in a way that I would have never imagined possible.

My stomach has probably been out of place since a stressful birth and with the addition of a few whiplashes and dental work it was something I had gotten use to. Yet after having a niacin overdose that rocked my world I started having heart palpitations that was effecting my sleep because my stomach was pressing against the pericardium. Having my stomach put back in place helped immensely. Being an energy healer I now am able to help many people with the knowledge imparted to me about Hiatal Hernia and the many symptoms that express themselves when the stomach is out of place such as acid reflux, pressure in the diaphragm and irritable bowel. Dr. Selinsky is a brilliant man with knowledge that should be taught to all medical students and doctors that would eliminate the need for anti-acids, indigestion and some cases of heart disease.

- Deborah Mills - Soul Focused Healer

The first time I went to Dr. Phil, I walked out of his room in awe. He answered so many questions for me. I loved his analogy of a car to a body. It simplified so many unanswered questions that I had. That was over two years ago. I originally went to him for a weight loss solution. He diagnosed me with a hiatal hernia. He was able to manipulate my stomach and manually pull it down. Since then it has never gone back up. I still continue to see him on a regular basis for my mental and physical health. He is a wonderful teacher and during our sessions he openly shares his knowledge and educates me on overall health and wellbeing. At the same time he manipulates my body, diagnosing the current condition of my liver, kidneys and other vital organs.

He is able to "re-set" my clock and I leave feeling like a million dollars. I have lost about 10 pounds over the last year, however, I realize that it's up to me to watch what I am eating, and that there is no magic pill.

- C. P. -

1.

Dr. Phil helped me with combating debilitating asthma. Since seeing him, I have had no more regular hospitalizations, recurring pneumonia, nor the need to return to go on prednisone. He has improved my overall immune system, energy, and has helped my body to repair the "damage" done by years of harsh medications. Dr. Phil has helped me to understand how the body works. No matter what questions I have regarding health concerns, he always has a clear explanation and logical natural solution.

2.

My brother was on disability for a huge infection in his feet and his legs up to the knees, both feet completely swollen from infection that stemmed from blisters below the foot calluses that broke open. He has no feeling in his toes (peripheral neuropathy), and that is why it had gotten so bad. His doctor said that the antibiotics were not working, and prepared him to have at least one toe amputated. Dr. Phil worked on my brother's entire body, performed the pressure needed to "de-herniate" his stomach, advised natural supplements, diet, and care of the feet. After the treatment, my brother felt energized for the first time in weeks. Within one week, the antibiotics started working (probably finally being absorbed properly), along with the additional supplements, and the redness and swelling went down tremendously. The next time he saw his doctor for a "pre-op" visit, the doctor could not believe the improvement, and opted not to amputate. After a two-month ordeal, he is back to work and well.
- Ruth Harper -

Doctor Selinsky,
Because of your knowledge of the human body and your homeopathic advice, I am living a healthy and productive life! Thank you for always being available to me and your patients, twenty four seven.
- Reid Hoshizaki - Harbor City, Ca

In file://localhost/message/%253C7C72A9B789544E25B9DB052F1A4 F50D3.MAI@apexenergetics.com%253E2008 my oldest daughter was diagnosed with pancreatic cancer. She suffered for two years with abdominal pains. As her mother, I was emotionally and energetically bonded with her. When she telephoned me and said, "Mom, I hurt", I felt her pain. I became nauseated every day. I lost 30 pounds and became weaker and weaker. My medical doctor told me that there was nothing wrong with me. He said, "It's all in your head". I went to a massage therapist who said she could not work on me because I was too nauseated.

She gave me the name of a person who had taught the physiology section of her massage classes. During the appointment, he assessed that my stomach was tucked up too high under my ribs. As I lay on the massage table, he literally pulled my stomach down. Dr. Phil Selinsky was the beginning of my recovery. I continued to see him weekly and followed his advice for health. I gradually regained some weight. My daughter continued her devastating decline. However, I was then strong enough to help her. She finally passed away in 2010. I am grateful to Dr. Phil Selinsky for helping me to attain a strong foundation for health. *– Letty Lauffer, PhD. -*

I have been a recipient of Dr. Phil's healing powers for over a year. I came to him with issues I had incurred at work. I was sent from Dr. to Dr. and given an elixir of different medications that were doing nothing to alleviate the pain or condition. I was experiencing the band-aid affect and realized this was as good as it was going to get. Their treatment was not going to fix the problem only mask the symptoms. I received an email about Dr. Phil's clinic and the way he views and understands the human body got my interest. I went to the clinic and was fascinated by his technique and healing style. I made an appointment to see him and the results have been amazing. Dr. Phil told me it would take some time to get everything back working again the way the body is supposed to, but I would need to be patient and things would get better. He was right and I have not been back to see a medical Dr. for a work injury or for that matter anything for quite sometime. My health and well-being have greatly improved and been corrected. I am so grateful for his dedication and understanding of the human body, it has made all the difference in my life. *- Mary Ann Porter -*

Dr. Phil Selinsky has a wonderful way of making complicated issues regarding the body and health clear and understandable. He seems to effortlessly communicate information regarding what he perceives to be the root causes of most "dis-eases." Perhaps more people will experience peace after reading his book by understanding their reactions and behaviors from deep physiological, emotional, psychological, and spiritual levels.
- Richelle (Ricky) Gaspar, MA, LMFT, SEP – Santa Barbara, Ca

APPENDIX II

REFERENCES

Baroody, Theodore D.C., N.D., *ALKALIZE OR DIE : Superior Health Through Proper Alkaline-Acid Balance* [Paperback] - Waynesville, N.C. - Holographic Health Press – (2002) | ISBN-10: 0961959533

Baroody, Theodore D.C., N.D., *HIATAL HERNIA SYNDROME : Insidious Link to Major Illness - A Guide to Self-Healing* - Waynesville, N.C. Holographic Health Press Inc (June 1987) 6th edition- ISBN-10: 0961959525 ISBN-13: 978-0961959524

Bernays, Edward L., Miller, Mark Crispin *PROPAGANDA* - Ig Publishing, (1928) ISBN: 0970312598, 9780970312594

Connelly, Dianne M., PhD. *TRADITIONAL ACUPUNCTURE: THE LAW OF THE 5-ELEMENTS* - Wisdomwell Press; 2nd edition (October 1, 1994) ISBN-10: 0912381035 ISBN-13: 978-0912381039

Deal, Sheldon, D.C., N.D. *NEW LIFE THROUGH NATURAL METHODS* Publisher, New Life, Tucson Arizona (1979)

Deal, Sheldon, D.C., N.D. *NEW LIFE THROUGH NUTRITION* - New Life Publishing Co. Tucson, Arizona (1974) ASIN: B000Y59CT6

Diamond, Harvey and Marilyn *FIT FOR LIFE* - Grand Central Life & Style Reprint edition; (August 16, 2010) ISBN-10: 0446553646 ISBN-13: 978-0446553643

Diamond, Harvey and Marilyn *FIT FOR LIFE* - Warner Books, Inc. 1st edition (1985) ISBN 0-446-51322-9

Eidem, William Kelley *THE DOCTOR WHO CURES CANCER* – Createspace (July 20, 2008) ISBN: 9781438263908

Goodheart, George, D.C., <www.anatomytrains.com> Copyright Kinesis, Inc. (2012)

Goodheart, George, D.C., <www.kinesiology.nu/courses/003.html>. This newsletter has been produced by Dr Donald McDowall of the Macquarie Chiropractic Clinic, Canberra Australia and is copyright to Cosmos Pty Ltd (1998,1999) (ACN 008 593 173)

Gray, Henry, F.R.S. *GRAY'S ANATOMY* - W.B. Saunders Co 36 edition (December 1980) ISBN-10: 0721691285 ISBN-13: 978-0721691282

Guyton, Arthur C., M.D. *TEXT BOOK OF MEDICAL PHYSIOLOGY* – W. B. Saunders Co 9th edition (January 15, 1996) ISBN-10: 0721659446 ISBN-13: 978-0721659442

Hamer, Ryke Geerd, M.D. *DOCUMENTS OF THE NEW MEDICINE* - Amici di Dirk (August 1, 2000) ISBN-10: 8493009199 ISBN-13: 9788493009199

Howell, Edward, D.C. *ENZYME NUTRITION* - Avery Publishing Group; 1St Edition (January 1, 1995) ISBN-10: 0895292211 ISBN-13: 978-0895292216

Kellogg, John Harvey, M.D. *COLON HYGIENE: COMPRISING NEW AND IMPORTANT FACTS CONCERNING THE PHYSIOLOGY OF THE COLON AND AN ACCOUNT OF PRACTICAL AND SUCCESSFUL METHODS OF COMBATING INTESTINAL INACTIVITY AND TOXEMIA* - Good Health Publishing Co. Battle Creek, Mich (1915)
<http://books.google.com/books?id=OmwPAAAAYAAJ&pg=PA7& lpg=PA7&dq=COLON+HYGIENE:+COMPRISING+NEW+AND+ IMPORTANT+FACTS+CONCERNING+THE+PHYSIOLOGY+ OF+THE+COLON+AND+AN+ACCOUNT+OF+PRACTICAL+ AND+SUCCESSFUL+METHODS+OF+COMBATING+

INTESTINAL+INACTIVITY+AND+TOXEMIA++Good+Health+
Publishing+Co.+Battle+Creek,+Mich+(1915)&source=bl&ots=qqyqb
ZL61E&sig=l5eX5ORcjmJI98qqkPkycg3Ez3I&hl=en&sa=X&ei=J_
0MUIL2LPH62AWEn4AL&ved=0CDcQ6AEwAQ#v=onepage&
q=COLON%20HYGIENE%3A%20COMPRISING%20NEW%
20AND%20IMPORTANT%20FACTS%20CONCERNING%20
THE%20PHYSIOLOGY%20OF%20THE%20COLON%20AND
%20AN%20ACCOUNT%20OF%20PRACTICAL%20AND%20
SUCCESSFUL%20METHODS%20OF%20COMBATING%20
INTESTINAL%20INACTIVITY%20AND%20TOXEMIA%20
%20Good%20Health%20Publishing%20Co.%20Battle%20Creek
%2C%20Mich%20(1915)&f=false>

Kellogg, John Harvey, M.D. *THE ART OF MASSAGE: A PRACTICAL MANUAL FOR THE NURSE, THE STUDENT AND THE PRACTITIONER* latest edition Kessinger Publishing, (2012) ISBN: 1169338291 / 1-169-33829-1

Kellogg, John Harvey, M.D. *THE ART OF MASSAGE: A PRACTICAL MANUAL FOR THE NURSE, THE STUDENT AND THE PRACTITIONER* - Modern Medicine Publishing Co., U.S.A., (1929) revised; Reprint (1975)

Loomis, Howard F., D.C. *ENZYMES: THE KEY TO GOOD HEALTH, VOL 1 (The Fundamentals)* Grote Pub (August 2005) ISBN-10: 0976912406 ISBN-13: 978-0976912408

Miehlke, K., M.D., Williams, R.M., M.D., Lopez, D.A., M.D. - *ENZYMES – THE FOUNTAIN OF L IFE* - Neville Press (August 1994) ISBN-10: 1884303005 ISBN-13: 978-1884303005

Pottenger Francis M. Jr., M.D. *POTTENGER'S CATS: A STUDY IN NUTRITION* - Price-Pottenger Fondation; 2nd edition (June 1, 1995) ISBN-13: 978-0916764067 ISBN-10: 0916764060

Price, Weston A., D.D.S. *NUTRITION AND PHYSICAL DEGENERATION* - Price-Pottenger Nutrition Foundation - 6th edition, 14th printing. La Mesa, CA, USA., 2000. ISBN 0-87983-816-7

Rogers, Sherry, M.D., *DETOXIFY OR DIE* - Sarasota, Florida, Sand Key Company, Inc. (December 1, 2002) ISBN-13: 9781887202046

Rogers, Sherry, M.D., *NO MORE HEARTBURN* - Publisher: New York, N.Y. Kensington Publishing Corp. (2000) ISBN-10: 1575665107 ISBN-13: 978-1575665108

Shelton, Herbert M., D.C., N.D. *FOOD COMBINING MADE EASY* - Book Pub Co. - latest edition (2012) ISBN: 9781570672606

Shelton, Herbert M., D.C., N.D. *FOOD COMBINING MADE EASY* - Willow Pub; 1st rev. print edition (June 1940) ISBN-10: 0960694803 ISBN-13: 978-0960694808

Shelton, Herbert M., D.C., N.D. *TOXEMIA* - Kessinger Publishing, LLC (September 15, 2006) ISBN-10: 1430424052 ISBN-13: 978-1430424055

Simoncini, Tullio, M.D. *CANCER IS A FUNGUS* Edizioni; 2nd edition (September 1, 2007) ISBN-10: 8887241082 ISBN-13: 978-8887241082

Stoner, Fred, D.C., N.D., *THE ECLECTIC APPROACH TO CHIROPRACTIC* - Las Vegas, Nevada, F.L.S. Publishing Co (1976) OL19294835M LCCN 98001899

Stone, Randolph, N.D., D.C., D.O., *Dr. Randolph Stone's Polarity Therapy: The Complete Collected Works* – Book Pub Co. (1999) ISBN-10 157067079X, ISBN-13 9781570670794

Thie, John, D.C. *TOUCH FOR HEALTH* – Santa Monica, California - Devorss & Co. (December, 1973) LCCCN 73-86019 ISBN 0-87516-180-4

Thie, John, D.C. *TOUCH FOR HEALTH* – Santa Monica, California - Devorss & Co. - New & Revised Edition (May, 2012) ISBN-10: 087516871X ISBN-13: 978-0875168715

Tye, Larry *THE FATHER OF SPIN: EDWARD L. BERNAYS AND THE BIRTH OF PUBLIC RELATIONS* - Picador (September 1, 2002) ISBN-10: 0805067892 ISBN-13: 978-0805067897

Varmus, Harold, M.D. *THE FUTURE OF CANCER RESEARCH: CHALLENGES AND OPPORTUNITIES* - Uploaded by AACRNews on Apr 3, 2011 Interview with Harold Varmus, M.D., director, National Cancer Institute <http://www.youtube.com/watch?v=JOAMegO9RWo>

Warburg, Otto H., M.D. *THE PRIME CAUSE AND PREVENTION OF CANCER* Revised lecture at the meeting of the Nobel Laureates on June 30, 1966 at Lindau, Lake Constance, Germany by Otto Warburg, Director, Max Planck-Institute for Cell Physiology, Berlin-Dahlem English Edition by Dean Burk, National Cancer Institute, Bethesda, Maryland, USA The Second Revised Edition Published by Konrad Triltsch, Würzburg, Germany, 1969 - Nobel Prize in medicine in 1931

Weinberg, Robert A., PhD. *GENES AND THE BIOLOGY OF CANCER* - Taylor & Francis, Inc. (May 2006) ISBN: 0815340761 ISBN-13: 9780815340768

Wong, William, N.D. PhD. *WHAT ARE SYSTEMIC ENZYMES AND WHAT DO THEY DO?* © Copyright 1999 Dr. William Wong and his licensors.

<http://www.totalityofbeing.com/FramelessPages/Articles/WhatAre SystemicEnzymes.htm>

Worsley, J.R. *5 – ELEMENT WORSLEY ACUPUNCTURE* - Redwing Book Co (January 1998) ISBN-10: 0788194526 ISBN-13: 978-0788194528

APPENDIX III

The following is a list of different types of health practitioners to help you choose the best help to fit your own specific health needs.

HEALTH PRACTITIONER DEFINITIONS

N.D. = Naturopathic Doctor
> Doctor = Teacher
> Naturopathic = Pathic (from pathos) = suffering
>> Naturo (from natural) = not man made - occurring In Nature
>> Treating suffering using Natural methods (a holistic approach using herbs, exercise, tissue manipulation, etc.)

M.D. = Medical Doctor
> (Allopathic "Western" Medicine)
>> Allo (from allos) = different/confrontational
>> Pathic (from pathos) = suffering
>> Treating suffering using confrontational methods (drugs and surgery)

Hm.D. = Doctor of Homeopathic Medicine
> (Most homeopaths are Medical Doctors) Homeo = same
>> Pathic (from pathos) = suffering
>> Treating suffering using miniscule doses of substances which would cause the presenting symptoms if taken in larger doses

D.O. = Doctor of Osteopathic Medicine
> Osteo (ostium) = bone
> Pathic (from pathos) = suffering
>> Treating suffering by manipulating bones and connective tissue (Osteopaths receive M.D. training plus manipulation)

D.C. = Doctor of Chiropractic Medicine

Chiro (from chiro) = hand

Practic (from practikos) = practice

Treating suffering using hand manipulations ("adjustments")

D.Ac. = Doctor of Acupuncture

("Eastern" Medicine)

Treating suffering by stimulating acupuncture points using needles, heat, cold, herbs, magnetics, electrical, finger pressure, stretching, exercise, etc. resulting in balance or homeostasis.

APPENDIX IV

LICENSE VS CERTIFICATION

License = a tax paid to a political entity for the privilege of doing business within its boundaries.

Certification = acknowledgement by an educational facility or agency of a proscribed level of education and/or achievement

The mere possession of a "license" does not imply expertise!

A license assures nothing other than the fact that you have paid a tax to a political subdivision. Typically, the enactment of a licensing law for any group or profession stems from a small number of individuals who want to limit their competition by insisting that any new arrivals to the activity or profession must pass rigorous requirements that the original group did not need to accomplish. The original group is now "protected" by the force of statute Law.

If you are looking for evidence of competency and expertise, you must check the "certification of competency" from a specific educational institution with a recognized reputation.

APPENDIX V

AUTHOR'S BIOGRAPHY

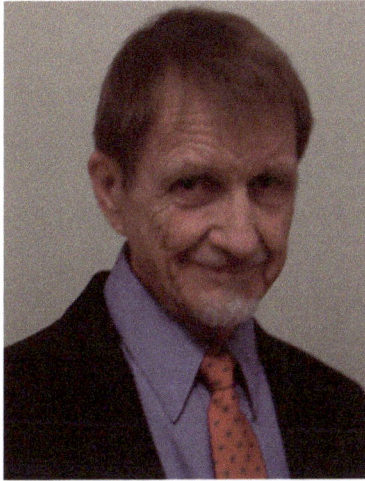

Phil Selinsky, N.D.

After almost 20 years in mechanical engineering designing automated machines and tools for GM, Ford, and Chrysler in Michigan, and McDonnel Douglas and Convair and Proctor & Gamble in California, Phil decided to apply his engineering skills to more complex machines (human bodies).

- He completed training as a Hypnotherapist from the Hypnosis Motivation Institute in 1974.
- He graduated from the Los Angeles College of Massage and Physical Therapy's Instructor Training Course in 1976.
- With the very creative help of Karen Halcyon, he founded the INSTITUTE FOR HOLISTIC STUDIES in Santa Barbara in 1976.

- He obtained the California Office of Private and Post Secondary Education approval for:
  The first 1000-hour Holistic Health Practitioner Program in the State of California
  The first massage instruction video program in California
  The first "approved" school of hypnosis in California.
- He created the first "Chair Massage" program, instruction book, and video program in California.
- He also founded the Central Coast Chapter of the American Massage Therapy Association (AMTA) and served as the Public Relations Director for the American Massage Therapy Association (California Chapter).
- He received his certification in Advanced Modern and Traditional Acupuncture from the Occidental Institute for Chinese Studies in 1979.
- He graduated from the Anglo-American Institute for Naturopathic Studies in 1980.
- He has also maintained a private Naturopathic practice in Santa Barbara, Thousand Oaks, Ojai, Glendora, and San Diego in addition to his teaching commitments over the past 35 years.
- He has taught a NATURAL HEALTH AND MASSAGE THERAPY class at the Santa Barbara Body Therapy Institute in Santa Barbara and an 18 credit hour NATURAL HEALING class at Citrus College in Glendora as well as a 100 hour FULL BODY REFLEX workshop at Pacific Beach Yoga and Healing Arts Center in San Diego.
- He is the author of the three-volume book series, "THE HUMAN MACHINE ... A Trouble Shooter's Manual" which approaches the question: What is the design purpose of this machine (our bodies)?
- He is also the co-author of the Amazon Best Selling Book "WIN – 35 Winning Strategies from Today's Leading Entrepreneurs" from *Celebrity Press*.

www.ingramcontent.com/pod-product-compliance
Lightning Source LLC
Chambersburg PA
CBHW040857210326
41597CB00029B/4881